SUPPLEMENT TO VOLUME 67, 1989, OF THE

BULLE[TIN]

OF THE WORLD HEALTH ORGANIZATION
DE L'ORGANISATION MONDIALE DE LA SANTE

THE SCIENTIFIC JOURNAL OF WHO • LA REVUE SCIENTIFIQUE DE L'OMS

INFANT FEEDING
THE PHYSIOLOGICAL BASIS

EDITED BY
JAMES AKRE

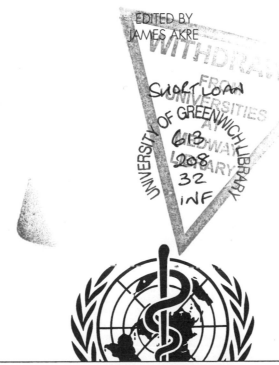

WORLD HEALTH ORGANIZATION, GENEVA • ORGANISATION MONDIALE DE LA SANTE, GENEVE

Reprinted (with corrections) 1992

Also available in French and Spanish

ISBN 92 4 068670 3
Printed in Belgium
89/8267 – Ceuterick – 8500
91/8749 – Ceuterick – 1500 (R)
91/8839 – Ceuterick – 2500 (R)
92/9336 – Ceuterick – 7500 (R)

CONTENTS

ACKNOWLEDGEMENTS

This review grew out of requests made by the World Health Assembly that WHO provide its Member States with up-to-date information concerning those rare circumstances in which infants cannot, or should not be breast-fed, and about the physiological development of the infant and its implications for complementary feeding. The original offset documents covering these topics, which form the basis for chapters 3 and 4 respectively, were prepared in 1985–86 by Dr Moises Behar, former Chief, Nutrition Unit, WHO, Geneva (present address: Tronco 8 L-22, El Encinal, Mixco III, Guatemala). Dr Behar was also instrumental in laying the groundwork for chapters 5 and 6, in addition to contributing to the overall conceptual framework that binds the review.

Special thanks are due to Maureen Minchin, lactation consultant, lecturer and author on infant feeding (address: 5 Saint George's Road, Armadale 3143, Australia), who contributed substantially to chapter 2 and reviewed other chapters for their technical accuracy and completeness; and to Dr Mary J. Renfrew, midwife and researcher (National Perinatal Epidemiology Unit, Radcliffe Infirmary, Oxford OX2 6HE, England), for her helpful suggestions.

The editor, James Akré, is Technical Officer in the Nutrition Unit, Division of Health Protection and Promotion, WHO, Geneva.

The contributions of the following persons to one or more chapters are also gratefully acknowledged:
—Dr Peter Aggett, Department of Child Health, University of Aberdeen, Foresterhill, Aberdeen AB9 2ZD, Scotland.
—Dr Peter Hartmann, Professor of Biochemistry, University of Western Australia, Perth, Western Australia, Australia.
—Dr Tahire Koçtürk-Runefors, Nutritionist and paediatrician, Mariehällsvägen 40, 18400 Akersberga, Sweden.
—Dr Felicity Savage, Senior Lecturer, Institute of Child Health, 30 Guildford Street, London W1, England.
—Dr Eberhard Schmidt, Director, Paediatric Clinic II, University of Düsseldorf, Moorenstrasse 5, Düsseldorf, Federal Republic of Germany.
—Dr A.M. Tomkins, Professor of Tropical Child Health, Institute of Child Health, 30 Guildford Street, London W1, England.

INTRODUCTION

Breast-feeding of human infants has been a common feature of all cultures and all times because our very survival has depended on it. In contrast, other modes of infant feeding—what is fed, when, how and by whom—have differed according to both time and place. Thus, various feeding customs have evolved through the ages by a process of trial and error, each one adapted to suit a given environment and often the best that could be expected nutritionally.

Breast-feeding was therefore a universal "natural imperative", ensuring infant survival and health. By the late nineteenth century, however, advances in science, especially biochemistry, led to new perceptions about the dietary needs of populations in the rapidly industrializing and urbanizing regions of Europe and North America. The challenges at this time included how to feed infants and young children safely, while avoiding dietary complications created by changes in life-styles, cultural values, and the roles of mothers and others responsible for child care.

During the early part of the twentieth century, and for many years thereafter, the emphasis in infant feeding reflected a primarily quantitative approach, which was considered more precise and therefore more "scientific". For example, analyses of human and cow's milk, although showing distinct differences, seemed to suggest that the latter could be safely modified to satisfy the nutritional needs of the infant. The first commercially produced breast-milk substitutes and complementary, or weaning, foods used as their model the then-available and very limited knowledge about the nutritional value of breast milk, and the physiology and nutritional needs of the newborn infant and young child. The basic criterion for the nutritional adequacy of these foods was growth, and not infrequently such notions as more food and earlier feeding became synonymous with better nutrition.

Today, it is clear that appropriate feeding practices during the first year of life are subject to a greater variety of considerations. The main factors are the infants' nutritional needs and degree of functional maturity, particularly as regards the type of food given, and their excretory processes and defences against infection. This review brings together the latest scientific information concerning the physiological development of infants during the prenatal period and first year of life and their implications for infant feeding. It describes why breast milk, which is naturally adapted to the evolving nutritional needs of young infants, is the only truly universal source of nourishment. It also shows

Parce qu'il s'agit de la survie de l'espèce, l'alimentation au sein des jeunes enfants a toujours été une des caractéristiques marquantes de toutes les cultures de tous les temps. A l'opposé, à part les pratiques relatives à l'allaitement au sein, ce que l'enfant mange, quand, comment et par qui la nourriture lui est offerte a varié grandement selon le temps et les situations géographiques. Les coutumes alimentaires ont indubitablement évolué à travers les âges grâce à un processus essais-erreurs et sur la base de l'expérience accumulée dans l'adaptation à des environnements donnés. Souvent, il s'agissait des meilleures coutumes possibles d'un point de vue nutritionnel dans les circonstances existantes.

L'allaitement maternel était donc un "impératif naturel" universel, jouant comme il l'a fait un rôle déterminant dans la santé et la survie de l'enfant. Cependant dès la fin du 19ème siècle, la science et particulièrement la biochimie avaient fait suffisamment de progrès pour entraîner une perception nouvelle de l'évolution des besoins diététiques des populations dans les régions rapidement urbanisées et industrialisées de l'Europe et de l'Amérique du Nord. Le défi tel qu'il était perçu à ce stade incluait la manière d'alimenter sainement les nourrissons et les jeunes enfants en évitant les complications diététiques créées par le développement de modes de vie non traditionnels, des changements dans les valeurs culturelles et des modifications du rôle des mères et d'autres responsables des soins aux enfants.

Durant la première partie du 20ème siècle et pendant de nombreuses années ensuite, l'accent mis sur l'alimentation infantile a reflété essentiellement une approche quantitative, qui était jugée plus précise et par conséquent plus "scientifique". Une analyse globale du lait humain et du lait de vache, bien que montrant de nettes différences, semblait suggérer que le dernier pouvait être aisément et sans danger modifié pour répondre aux besoins nutritionnels de l'enfant. Les premiers substituts et compléments du lait maternel produits commercialement utilisèrent comme base la connaissance— relativement grossière et limitée—que l'on avait à l'époque de la valeur nutritionnelle du lait humain et de la physiologie et des besoins nutritionnels du nouveau-né et du jeune enfant. Le critère pour évaluer la valeur nutritionnelle de ces aliments était basé sur la croissance et bien souvent des notions telles que plus d'aliments plus tôt étaient synonymes de meilleure nutrition.

Aujourd'hui, il est clair que durant la première année de la vie des pratiques alimentaires that later in the first year of life when other foods become necessary, these can be as varied as family diets around the world. What is essential is that the nutritional requirements should be met; the wider the range of foods eaten the easier this will be. Even at this stage of infant development, breast milk still provides a significant source of energy and nutrients as well as protection against infection and disease.

This review provides the scientific basis for preparing guidelines on infant feeding, taking into account the available foods and local customs. It is intended mainly for general practitioners, obstetricians, paediatricians, midwives, nutritionists and nurses, and for those in schools of public health; it will also be of interest to general readers who wish to update their knowledge of the subject.

Finally, a number of practical indications are presented in three annexes. Annex 1 is a check-list for evaluating the adequacy of support for breast-feeding provided in maternity hospitals, wards and clinics; it is taken from a joint WHO/UNICEF statement on this subect, which was published in 1989. Annex 2 suggests an empirical framework for studying the weaning process, which is an important first step in designing, carrying out and evaluating the impact of programmes intended to improve the nutritional status of infants and young children. Annex 3 suggests titles for further reading in this area, including selected WHO publications, and sources of information and learning materials.

appropriées doivent prendre en compte des considérations nettement plus subtiles et variées. Les principaux déterminants sont les besoins nutritionnels du nourrisson et son degré de maturité fonctionnelle, singulièrement en ce qui concerne le type d'aliments donnés et les capacités d'excrétion et de défense contre l'infection. C'est dans ce contexte que cette revue rassemble l'information scientifique la plus récente sur le développement physiologique de l'enfant durant la période prénatale et la première année de la vie avec les implications que cela entraîne sur l'alimentation. On décrit les raisons pour lesquelles le lait maternel, parce qu'il est naturellement adapté aux besoins physiologiques évolutifs du nourrisson, est la seule nourriture vraiment universelle. On démontre aussi que plus tard dans la première année de la vie, quand d'autres aliments deviennent nécessaires, ils peuvent être aussi variés que tous les régimes familiaux que l'on rencontre dans le monde. Ce qui est essentiel c'est que les besoins nutritionnels soient couverts et plus l'éventail d'aliments offerts est grand plus les chances sont meilleures qu'ils le soient. Cependant, même à ce stade du développement infantile le lait maternel constitue encore une source énergétique et nutritive significative en plus de son rôle protecteur contre la maladie.

Cette revue fournit les bases scientifiques pour l'élaboration des guides diététiques pour l'alimentation infantile en prenant en compte les coutumes locales et les aliments disponibles. Elle est principalement destinée aux médecins généralistes, aux obstétriciens, aux pédiatres, aux sages-femmes, aux nutritionnistes et aux infirmières, et aux écoles de santé publique. Elle intéressera aussi bien les lecteurs du grand public qui voudraient mettre à jour leurs connaissances sur le sujet.

Enfin, un certain nombre d'informations d'ordre pratique sont présentées dans trois annexes. L'annexe 1 est une liste de contrôle pour l'évaluation de la pertinence avec laquelle l'allaitement maternel est encouragé dans les services liés à la maternité; elle est empruntée à une déclaration conjointe OMS/UNICEF sur le sujet, publiée en 1989. L'annexe 2 propose un cadre empirique pour l'étude du sevrage, ce qui est une étape importante dans la formulation, la mise en oeuvre et l'évaluation de l'impact de programmes destinés à améliorer l'état nutritionnel des nourrissons et des jeunes enfants. L'annexe 3 suggère des références complémentaires sur la question, y compris certaines publications de l'OMS ainsi que différents matériels éducatifs et d'information.

1. The prenatal and immediate postpartum periods

A mother's nutritional status during pregnancy has important implications for both her own health and her ability to produce and breast-feed a healthy infant. Knowledge about adequate maternal nutrition during pregnancy is incomplete, however, and there is still considerable debate about the level of extra energy needed by a pregnant woman. A woman's usual nutritional requirements increase during pregnancy to meet her needs and those of the growing fetus. Additional energy is needed because of increased basal metabolism, the greater cost of physical activity, and the normal accumulation of fat as the energy reserve. The protein, vitamin and mineral requirements of the mother also increase during pregnancy, but the precise amounts for the last two are still a matter for discussion. A woman's weight increments during pregnancy vary between privileged and underprivileged communities. In addition to calcium, phosphorus and iron, a mother provides considerable amounts of protein and fat for fetal growth. Placental metabolism and placental blood flow, which are interrelated, are the most critical factors for fetal development.

The nutritional requirements of healthy newborns vary widely according to their weight, gestational age, rate of growth, as well as environmental factors. However, recommendations for some components may be derived from the average composition of early human milk and the amounts consumed by healthy, mature newborns who are following a normal postpartum clinical course. The water requirements of infants are related to their caloric consumption, activity, rate of growth, and the ambient temperature. A postnatal weight loss of 5–8% of body weight is usual during the first few days of life in mature newborn infants; in contrast, infants who experienced intrauterine malnutrition lose little or no weight at all.

The dynamic process of mother–newborn interaction from the first hours of life is intimately related to successful early breast-feeding. If this process is delayed, however, it may take longer and may be more difficult to achieve. Close mother–infant contact immediately after birth also helps infants to adapt to their new unsterile environment. Because drugs can interfere with bonding and breast-feeding, such substances should be given only when necessary and their effects should be evaluated. In general, young infants, especially newborns, have very irregular feeding intervals. It is advisable for numerous reasons to feed them whenever they indicate a need.

Introduction

The dual focus of this chapter—meeting the nutritional needs of the fetus at minimal cost to the mother and ensuring immediate and appropriate postpartum mother–child interaction—may appear disparate at first glance. However, as will become clear, these aspects are intimately related, critical as they are to promoting maternal and child health. The first influences pregnancy outcome, even as it protects the mother's nutritional status, while the second is paramount for the successful initiation and establishment of breast-feeding. In the 12-month period covered by this and the following chapters, both themes represent key first steps for the newborn infant on the road to a healthy productive life.

Nutritional aspects

The energy cost of pregnancy

A mother's nutritional status during pregnancy has important implications for both her own health and her ability to produce and breast-feed a healthy infant. Knowledge about what is adequate maternal nutrition during pregnancy is incomplete, and there is still considerable debate over the level of energy intake needed by a pregnant woman (1). For example, not enough is known about the metabolic alterations that occur, or their timing during pregnancy, or about when the mother builds up energy and nutrient stores for the growing fetus, and when her uterus, breasts, and blood and other bodily fluids are undergoing changes. Nor is it sufficiently clear how a pregnant woman, by regulating her physical activity, compensates for increased energy requirements and the rise in her basal metabolic rate. One has only to compare current dietary intake recommendations in many industrialized countries with the situation for most women in developing countries (2) to appreciate how incomplete the research on this subject is.

Results of recent longitudinal studies, which use more direct methods, are beginning to be published, however. For example, an integrated study conducted in the Gambia, Netherlands, Philippines, Scotland and Thailand showed that the energy costs of pregnancy were not met by anything like an equivalent energy intake. On this basis, the investigators concluded that both the 1981 Joint FAO/

WHO/UNU Expert Consultation's recommendation that women increase their food intake to supply an extra 1.0 MJ (240 kcal)/day (3) and the 1987 recommendation for women in Scotland of 1.2 MJ (285 kcal)/day (4) were not realistic for healthy populations living in industrialized countries.

In the Philippines, the findings seemed to suggest that pregnancy outcome can be successful despite a marginal energy intake (5), while the Gambian women studied appeared to be the beneficiaries of a remarkable physiological adjustment. By becoming pregnant the latter group saved so much energy in basal metabolism that they ended with a positive energy balance over the whole of pregnancy of about 46 MJ (11 000 kcal) (5).

The overall conclusion from these studies—that the total energy cost of pregnancy is about 250 MJ (60 000 kcal)—suggests that the recommendation in the FAO/WHO/UNU report was a full 25% too high. Even more striking is the fact that the extra 250 MJ of energy was not usually consumed in the diet (5). In another inquiry using the same protocol designed for the integrated study, the total energy cost of pregnancy for 57 healthy Dutch women was calculated to be 285 MJ (68 000 kcal) (6).

Because of steady advances in knowledge, including data from the five-country integrated study just cited, the recommendations of successive international expert groups differ in often important respects. Just as the intake-level recommended by the 1981 Consultation was lower than that of the 1971 Committee, it appears certain that future recommendations will be different again as the results of current studies become known. The information presented here is therefore part of a still-evolving picture of the real energy cost of pregnancy.

Nutritional requirements during pregnancy

A woman's normal nutritional requirements increase during pregnancy to meet the needs of the growing fetus and of the maternal tissues associated with pregnancy. Additional energy is also needed to meet the increased basal metabolism, the greater cost of physical activity, and the normal accumulation of fat as the energy reserve. The total additional energy needed for a normal pregnancy has been estimated to be about 335 MJ (80 000 kcal) over the nine-month period (3) but, as just discussed, this figure is now considered unrealistic. How much of this extra energy needs to be supplied by the diet is not clear and varies according to specific circumstances. As stated earlier, there are a number of metabolic adaptations whereby pregnant women can use dietary energy more efficiently. The amount of physical activity during pregnancy will also have a significant influence on energy needs; some women reduce their

physical activity while others continue to do hard physical labour. The nutritional status at the outset of pregnancy is also an important factor; obese women will not need to accumulate extra fat while thin women will.

A proper dietary balance is necessary to ensure sufficient energy intake for adequate growth of the fetus without drawing on the mother's own tissues to maintain her pregnancy. It has been shown, for example, that well-nourished women who eat a varied, balanced diet, and maintain a low level of physical activity, can have a normal pregnancy, gain adequate weight and produce healthy babies without any significant change in their pre-pregnancy dietary intake (3). On the other hand, chronically malnourished women with marginally adequate or frankly insufficient diets, who, in addition, continue to engage in heavy physical labour, usually gain very little weight during pregnancy, produce low-birthweight infants and experience a deterioration in their own nutritional status. Two classic studies, one conducted in Colombia (64) and the other in Guatemala (65), demonstrated the significant positive impact on birth weight, stillbirths, and neonatal and perinatal mortality of food supplementation of pregnant mothers at risk of malnutrition.

It was previously thought that the increased energy need was greater towards the end of pregnancy when fetal growth is significant. However, it has been found that, under normal circumstances, fat begins to accumulate from the outset of pregnancy in order to meet later needs for extra energy, particularly during lactation. It is thus recommended that the extra energy required during pregnancy should be distributed throughout the whole period. The FAO/WHO/UNU Consultation on Energy and Protein Requirements (3) recommended, under normal conditions, the addition of 1200 kJ (285 kcal)/day during pregnancy. If women are well nourished and reduce their physical activity during pregnancy, this extra allowance can be reduced to 200 kcal (840 kJ) per day. While these may prove to be overestimates of what is necessary for good pregnancy outcomes, it is clearly advisable, if at all possible, to increase the energy allowance for undernourished women in order to ensure significant fat deposits or at least to avoid further deterioration in their own nutritional status. Weight gain during pregnancy is a good indicator for regulating energy intake.

Protein intake is also critical during pregnancy. The extra protein needed for a woman who gains 12.5 kg during pregnancy and who produces a 3.3 kg infant has been estimated to be an average of about 3.3 g/day throughout pregnancy (3). The amount is low at the beginning and increases as pregnancy progresses; it needs to be corrected, however, according to the efficiency with which dietary protein is converted into tissue protein. The 1981 FAO/WHO/ UNU consultation recommended 6 g of extra protein/day throughout pregnancy if the protein comes from a varied diet containing foods of animal origin, which permit a margin of safety to cover individual variations.

Unlike energy, dietary protein surpluses do not accumulate. Women in well-to-do societies on usual diets frequently consume more protein than is actually required. Under these circumstances, the extra needs of pregnancy are met with no significant changes in dietary intake. However, for chronically undernourished women, for whom not only the total amount of dietary protein but also its biological value is frequently low, corrections during pregnancy are important. The addition of even small amounts of protein of high biological value (e.g., most proteins of animal origin) can enhance utilization of total dietary proteins and therefore significantly improve nutritional status. In order to prevent any protein imbalance in populations consuming varied diets, including proteins, but where the total energy intake is low, additional energy needs for pregnancy should be provided by an increase in the overall diet and not simply by the addition of starches or fats.

Vitamin and mineral requirements also increase during pregnancy, but the precise amount is still a matter for discussion. With balanced diets which satisfy the normal requirements of adult women for these nutrients, the extra intake needed to compensate for increased energy requirements during pregnancy should also, under normal conditions, cover the needed extra allowance of vitamins and minerals. An exception might be iron, in which women are frequently deficient even when they are otherwise well nourished (7). Significant amounts of additional iron are needed during pregnancy—about 1000 mg in all (8); however, this need is not equally distributed over the duration of pregnancy, the iron requirements of the fetus being most important during the second and third trimesters (8). Requirements during this period cannot be satisfied by dietary iron alone, even if it is of high bioavailability. Unless stores of about 500 mg exist before pregnancy, administration of iron supplements may be indicated if impairment of the expected increase in haemoglobin mass in the mother is to be avoided (8). It is still preferable, to the extent possible, to increase iron intake from dietary sources, as medicinal iron supplements have been reported to cause marked decreases in serum zinc levels (see chapter 2). Factors known to stimulate absorption of non-haem iron are the presence in the diet of meat, poultry, seafood and various organic acids, particularly ascorbic acid. On the other hand, a large number of substances, for example, polyphenols including tannins, phytates, certain forms of protein, and some forms of dietary fibre impair the absorption of non-haem iron (8).

When a diet is already deficient, even marginally, in some minerals or vitamins, the situation can become critical during pregnancy. For example, iodine-deficient populations suffer a variety of consequences that include goitre, low birth weight (see chapter 5), reduced mental function, and widespread lethargy. Irreversible forms of severe mental and neurological impairment, commonly known as cretinism, are observed in marked deficiency states (9). Similarly, in areas where there is a deficiency of vitamin A or thiamine, pregnant women and their infants are at risk.

Weight increments during pregnancy

Weight increments during pregnancy vary between privileged and underprivileged communities; the average weight gain, by the time of pregnancy, for mothers in the former group are given in Table 1.1.

Table 1.1: **Average weight gain during pregnancy in industrialized countries**[a]

Time of pregnancy (weeks)	Weight gain (kg)
1–12	0
13–20	2.4
21–24	1.5
25–28	1.9
29–32	2.0
33–36	2.0
37–40	1.2
Total:	10–12

[a] Reference 10.

A considerable proportion of weight gained during pregnancy is composed of protein and fat. Pregnant women in underprivileged communities normally have a much lower weight increment during pregnancy than women who are materially well off; if they do not have an adequate energy intake, they are more likely to lose fat and are at greater risk of giving birth to infants with low birth weight (2) (see chapter 5). It may be assumed that a reduction of fat deposits during pregnancy points to severe dietary deficiencies; however, an increase in fatty tissue, which is usual in affluent communities, may not be essential for a normal pregnancy outcome. The fat deposited during pregnancy is of great value, however, in compensating for the high energy requirements during lactation. If these reserves are not available, a mother's own tissues may be used to the detriment of her nutritional status.

Nutrient transfers during pregnancy

Nutrient transfers from mother to fetus are shown in Table 1.2. By the end of pregnancy the fetus has drawn about 30 g of calcium, 17 g of phosphorus and 300 mg of iron. At the same time, sizable amounts of minerals, which had been used in uterus and breast development, become available for meeting maternal nutritional needs.

Table 1.2: **Substances transferred to the fetus and placenta during pregnancy**[a]

	Newborn (g)	Placenta and amniotic fluid (g)
Total weight	3500	1450
Water	2530	1350
Protein	410	40
Fat	480	4
Sodium	5.7	3.9
Potassium	6.4	1.1
Chloride	6.0	3.1
Calcium	29.0	0.2
Phosphorus	16.9	0.6
Magnesium	0.8	0.06
Iron	0.3	0.01

[a] Reference 11.

Changes in maternal metabolism that promote adequate fetal growth

In addition to calcium, phosphorus and iron, a mother provides considerable amounts of protein and fat to promote adequate fetal growth. Since the transfer of most of these substances occurs most actively towards the third trimester, supplies of them have to be made available in time. This implies a biphasic cycle of the mother's intermediary metabolism, which is steered by endocrine influences during pregnancy (12). The energy balance of maternal tissues is assumed to be positive during the first half of pregnancy, which has been suggested by an apparent reduction in 3-methylhistidine excretion in the first part of pregnancy (13). This anabolic phase, with increased protein synthesis and an increase in fat tissue, is followed by catabolic processes characterized by a rapid formation of fetal tissues and depletion of maternal stores, which is not covered by the mother's usual nutrient intake (14,15). This process continues during lactation. The fetus, which has some of the characteristics of a parasite inside the maternal organism, is well protected by maternal nutrient stores. The stores compensate for seasonal variations in dietary intake and are activated through hormonal changes during pregnancy. The fetus is also protected by the active transport capacities of the placenta, which is able to mobilize nutrients, vitamins and minerals against concentration gradients in favour of the fetus (16).

The placenta

Placental function and fetal growth

Appropriate growth and development of the fetus is dependent on the functioning of the placenta. There are four areas of major importance (17): substrate and hormone concentrations in maternal circulation; uteroplacental blood flow; placental transfer mechanisms; and placental metabolism.

Substrate and hormone concentrations. Glucose is the main fuel for fetal metabolism (18), and its placental uptake is dependent on maternal blood glucose concentration (19). This does not apply to amino acids (20), but there is some correlation as regards free fatty acids (FFA). Placental hormones are able to regulate metabolic processes by modulating maternal substrate concentrations through changing the action of insulin on maternal tissues or regulating the mobilization of maternal plasma FFA (21). It is thus possible to direct glucose to the fetus in later pregnancy by lowering the insulin sensitivity in maternal tissue.

Uteroplacental blood flow. Near term, the uteroplacental blood flow ranges from 500 to 700 ml/minute (22). Little is known about earlier phases of pregnancy. Augmentation of uterine vessels, increase in maternal cardiac output, and increase of uterine vascular resistance are the basis for transfer of oxygen and amino acids to the fetus (23). Placental glucose uptake is severely reduced only when the blood flow is similarly restricted (24); maternal hypotension is thus considered a threat for fetal growth (25).

Placental transfer mechanisms. There are three main transfer mechanisms across the placenta (16): passive diffusion, dependent on blood flow; carrier-mediated facilitated diffusion; and active transport against concentration gradients, which is an energy-consuming process.

Glucose is transported by facilitated diffusion (26). Amino acids apparently are moved by active transport because their concentration in fetal blood is higher; there is selective transport for the neutral amino acids, whereas others (glutamic and aspartic acid) are not taken up (26). There is a gradient-dependent transport for FFA, although FFA in fetal and maternal blood are related. The process of maturation of the placenta, with marked reduction in the diameter of placental membranes in the course of pregnancy, may enhance diffusion and transport mechanisms.

Placental metabolism

The placenta, especially the trophoblast, is a very active metabolic tissue (17). Only 30–40% of glucose taken up by the placenta is transferred to the fetus, the rest being retained in the placental tissues (17), which are well equipped with insulin receptors (27). Moreover, lactate production represents about 40% of placental glucose utilization, lactate not being excreted into the human fetal circulation. Less is known about lipid metabolism of the placenta; the maternal hypertriglyceridaemia of late pregnancy may thus enhance an increased FFA uptake by the fetus (28). Amino-acid concentrations in the placenta exceed maternal and fetal values (29), a considerable proportion of which is returned to the maternal circulation as ammonia. Protein synthesis within the placenta essentially concerns hormone synthesis, especially of insulin receptors (27). The physiological role of placental insulin receptors has not been entirely clarified.

Placental metabolism and placental blood flow, which are interrelated, are the most critical factors for fetal development. The placenta is apparently able to adjust maternal metabolism to meet the needs of fetal growth through hormone synthesis.

The newborn

Nutritional requirements

Nutritional requirements of healthy newborns vary widely according to weight, gestational age, rate of growth and environmental factors. If one looks at breast-milk intake, the great variability of volume and composition during the immediate postpartum period does not lend itself to making recommendations based solely on breast-milk flow (30). However, recommendations for a few components may be derived from what is currently known about the average composition of early human milk, and the amounts consumed by healthy, mature newborns who are following a normal postpartum clinical course.

Where minor and trace elements in breast milk are concerned, the WHO study (31) on these elements that was conducted in Guatemala, Hungary, Nigeria, Philippines, Sweden and Zaire concluded that environmental conditions appear to play a major role in determining the concentration of most of them. However, for some of the elements (calcium, chlorine, magnesium, phosphorus, potassium and

sodium) there appeared to be little difference between groups and countries, and concentrations were not significantly influenced by maternal nutritional status.

The ranges of concentrations found under usual conditions, i.e., after excluding study areas where exceptionally low or high values were observed, may be useful in determining the desirable concentration of trace elements in breast-milk substitutes. The study also concluded, however, that it may be opportune to reconsider the recommendation of a WHO Expert Committee in 1973 (32) that infant formula should contain all the minor and essential trace elements, at least as much as is present in human milk. The emphasis at the time was on meeting minimum nutritional requirements. Today there is concern that infant formula contains levels of some trace elements far exceeding the normal nutritional requirements of infants during the first months of life. Breast-milk composition and maternal dietary needs for lactation are discussed further in chapter 2.

The water requirements of infants are related to caloric consumption, ambient temperature, activity, and rate of growth. Specific gravity of urine is influenced by the way the infant is fed. Breast-fed infants have a low solute load and therefore a low urine specific gravity, while the opposite is true for infants fed on breast-milk substitutes. Average water requirements for a healthy infant under normal environmental conditions are given in Table 1.3, while Table 1.4 shows the dependency of the water requirement in relation to the specific gravity of urine.

Table 1.3: **Average water requirements for infants**[a]

Age	Weight (kg)	Water (ml/kg)
3 days	3.0	80–100
10 days	3.2	125–150
3 months	5.4	140–160

[a] Reference 33.

Table 1.4: **Average water requirements of a 3-kg infant**[a]

Urine specific gravity	Volume		
	ml	ml/100 kcal	ml/kg
1.005	650	217	220
1.015	339	113	116
1.020	300	100	100
1.030	264	88	91

[a] Reference 33.

These figures are divided up as follows: 30 ml as skin loss, 50 ml through the respiratory tract, and 50–70 ml/100 kcal for excretion of non-concentrated urine. Infants fed only breast milk require no additional water, even in very hot climates (34), unless another, high-osmotic food is given, unless they lose excessive volumes of water due to diarrhoea, or unless they become severely overheated. In such cases, a small quantity of water given by cup or spoon will ease the infants irritability due to thirst. However, giving water regularly may decrease the frequency and intensity of breast-feeding, or inappropriately condition the infant's oral behaviour, with a consequent negative impact on breast-milk production and removal. Moreover, water may be contaminated in some environments or the feeding bottles may be a source of infection (35). In addition, water will dilute the protective effects and nutritional value of breast milk, and is associated with higher levels of neonatal jaundice (36).

Neonatal weight loss

A postnatal weight loss of 5–8% of body weight is usual during the first few days of life in mature newborn infants. Postnatal weight loss is the result of a fall of intracellular fluid after birth, particularly from the skin, and is influenced by feeding practice, humidity, ambient temperature and, to some degree, loss of meconium. In contrast, infants who experienced intrauterine malnutrition, i.e., who are small for gestational age, lose little or no weight at all. There is a shift to the extracellular compartment, which stabilizes after the third day, when intracellular water content begins to rise to its previous level. Infants mobilize and excrete water and electrolytes in the fasting state. Since plasma osmolarity remains stable, there may be a shift of sodium from intracellular to extracellular space (37). The provision of water during this phase accelerates losses (38). It is known from animal experiments that low fluid intake leads to retention of cell water, while high intake speeds its release (39). This is particularly critical in the case of premature infants who tend to retain considerable amounts of intracellular water when fluid intake is restricted. See chapter 5.

Other postpartum concerns

Importance of immediate contact between mother and infant after birth. The importance of the immediate postpartum period for healthy child development has been clarified through scientific investigation since the 1960s. This research began on the assumption that this is an "imprinting" period, a critical and sensitive early phase concerned with sudden and lasting attachment between the infant and the mother. The phenomenon was first observed in animals (40,41), and it was further postulated that this reaction existed for human mothers and their infants (42–45). The father can also contribute to this early bonding period; although his direct influence is usually limited, it is nevertheless significant given the impact his reaction can have on the mother (46).

The immediate initiation and evolution of the parent–newborn interaction is structured by a mother's life experience and her conscious and unconscious attitudes. In the dynamic process which begins at birth, neonates are by no means as passive as their limited development may suggest (47). Most of the many interactions between a mother and her infant in the first hours of life are closely related to successful early breast-feeding. Immediate contact may be provided initially and most effectively by placing the infant on the mother's abdomen, even before the umbilical cord has been clamped (48). Another way is to place the infant at the mother's side, facing the mother. Both facilitate the touching and eye-to-eye contact that play such an important role in a mother's own sense of satisfaction (49).

The immediate postnatal period is obviously not the only moment when attachment can develop; if the process is delayed, however, it may take longer and be more difficult to achieve. The classic studies have shown that immediate contact between mother and infant after birth positively influences attachment behaviour where fondling, kissing, looking in the face, and talking to the infant are concerned; later, with regard to frequency of picking up, increased proximity, and greater soothing in stress situations; and still later, as concerns effectiveness of speech contact (43,45). Notwithstanding the scepticism recently shown about the long-term effects of early contact (50,51), there is no doubt about its positive influence on the successful initiation and establishment of lactation (see chapter 2). However, it is important in this regard to distinguish between early contact without suckling and early contact that includes unrestricted suckling.

In addition to contributing to early attachment, close mother–infant contact immediately after birth also helps infants to adapt to their new unsterile environment by favouring colonization of their skin and gastrointestinal tract with their mothers' microorganisms. These tend to be non-pathogenic, and mothers' milk supplies antibodies specific for them. Infants are thus simultaneously exposed to, and protected against, the organisms for which active immunity will be developed only later in life.

Effects of anaesthesia or drugs on the infant postpartum.
In view of the significance of early mother–infant contact for successful breast-feeding, it is important to understand that drugs administered during labour may interfere with this process (52). Eye-opening by the infant after delivery may be delayed, thus affecting interaction between mother and child. Even very small doses of drugs can have serious consequences for an infant's neurobehaviour pattern and therefore on the quality of the early mother–neonate relationship (53). Drugs given to the mother may negatively influence feeding ability and nutrient intake in newborn infants for many days after delivery owing to the dependence of the fetus on maternal detoxification, and on the infant's drug excretion, which is slowed because of immaturity of the liver (54). The effects of obstetrical analgesia or anaesthesia on neonatal feeding behaviour have been reviewed elsewhere (55).

In pregnancy and during birth, most drugs pass easily from mother to fetus through the placental barrier. Analgesics, tranquillizers and other drugs affecting the central nervous system pass rapidly because the blood–brain interchange has the same characteristics as the placental barrier. Changes in the reactions of newborn infants under the influence of various drugs have been observed as regards sleep and wakefulness, attentiveness to visual stimuli, oral behaviour in response to auditory and tactile stimuli, application of various neurobehavioural scales, ability to breast-feed well 24 hours after birth, and EEG patterns. Drugs that have been tested included pethidine (56,57) tranquillizers, barbiturates (53,58), and morphine derivatives (57); all affect the neonate's physiological state. Various investigations have also shown that even spinal anaesthetics given to the mother change the infant's neurobehavioural status (55), although this may be partly due to premedications.

Because drugs can interfere with both attachment and breast-feeding, drugs should be given only when necessary and their effects should be evaluated. The application of antibiotic, or possibly silver nitrate, eye drops to prevent conjunctivitis in the infant is reported to delay immediate eye-to-eye contact (59). Where these drugs are still considered necessary their administration can be postponed for a time to allow eye-to-eye contact immediately after birth (60). See also chapter 3 for a discussion of drug therapy during lactation, and Annex 1.

The newborn infant's feeding

As will be discussed more fully in chapter 2, it is one of the more striking neurological capabilities of the newborn infant to be able to breast-feed vigorously within the first two hours after birth, even at gestational ages when bottle-feeding is difficult. In general young infants, especially newborns, have very irregular feeding intervals. They may feed at unevenly spaced intervals from 6 to 12, or as many as 18, times in a 24-hour period. Mothers may need reassurance that this early phase of very frequent feeding is likely to settle into more predictable routines as lactation is established. Indeed, lactation will be more speedily established if the mother and baby are encouraged to feed as often and as long as the infant wishes to do so. Correct positioning of the infant is important to prevent nipple trauma.

It is advisable for numerous reasons (61,62) to feed young infants whenever they indicate a need. Mothers can usually rely on their infants, who regulate their appetite well, to know when they have had enough to drink. To an experienced observer, the infant's clinical state and behavioural patterns before and after a feed will also indicate satiety or hunger. Mothers may need to be cautioned not to interpret an infant's possible unsettled behaviour as due to milk insufficiency (see chapter 3); there are many other possible causes. It is not advisable to weigh an infant before and after every feed. Daily weighing will usually be adequate during the first few days of life to monitor milk intake where this is thought to be necessary. Weekly weighing will be sufficient in the first weeks after birth to detect any possible nutritional problem early enough for appropriate action to be taken (63). Where relevant, catch-up growth can be extremely rapid during this period, even for infants who have failed to thrive for some weeks before a corrective intervention is begun.

Résumé

La période prénatale et les post-partum immédiat

Le statut nutritionnel de la mère durant la grossesse influe directement sur son état de santé et sur ses possibilités de donner naissance à un enfant sain qu'elle pourra allaiter. On ignore encore exactement la valeur des besoins énergétiques supplémentaires à couvrir pour une femme enceinte. On connaît mal les modifications métaboliques qui surviennent et le moment où elles se situent. De quelle manière la future mère en réglant son activité physique compense-t-elle l'augmentation de son métabolisme de base et ses besoins caloriques accrus?

Les résultats d'enquêtes longitudinales récentes utilisant des méthodes directes, conduites en Gambie, Hollande, Philippines, Ecosse et Thaïlande montrent que les coûts énergétiques de la grossesse ne sont pas compensés par une consommation énergétique équivalente. Sur ces bases les chercheurs ont constaté que les conclusions de la consultation d'experts conjointe FAO/OMS/UNU de 1981 qui recommandaient un accroissement de la ration fournissant 1.0 MJ/j, et les recommandations pour l'Ecosse de 1.2 MJ/j, n'étaient pas réalistes pour des populations en bonne santó dos pays industrialisés. Aux Philippines, certaines constatations suggèrent que le produit de la grossesse peut être tout à fait satisfaisant avec des apports énergétiques mineurs. De même des femmes en Gambie ont démontré des capacités remarquables d'adjustements physiologiques grâce à une adaptation à la grossesse de leur métabolisme de base. La conclusion de ces études est que l'on peut fixer le coût énergétique total de la grossesse à environ 250 MJ (60 000 kcal), soit un chiffre inférieur aux recommandations FAO/OMS/UNU. Ce qui est étonnant cependant c'est le fait que le fait que les femmes enceintes aient besoin de 250 MJ supplémentaires ne se traduise pas nécessairement par une augmentation de 250 MJ apportés par leur régime alimentaire.

Sont ensuite successivement envisagés:

—*Le gain de poids pendant la grossesse.* Il existe une différence entre pays en développement et pays industrialisés. La variation porte principalement sur les réserves en graisses. Dans les pays en développement les femmes se situent bien souvent en dessous des 10 à 12 kg de gain de poids généralement accepté.

—*Modifications du métabolisme maternel favorisant la croissance fœtale.* Les échanges les plus actifs en protéines, graisses, Ca, P et Fe se produisent durant le troisième trimestre de la grossesse; en conséquence la mère doit avoir constitué des réserves durant les deux premiers trimestres. L'équilibre énergétique maternel est positif durant la première moitié de la grossesse, du moins en ce qui concerne les protéines comme cela a été démontré par l'étude de l'excrétion de la méthyl-histidine.

—*Les besoins nutritionnels durant la grossesse.* Les recommandations FAO/OMS/UNU fixaient à 3.3 g de protéines supplémentaires par jour la ration pour une femme qui aurait pris 12.5 kg pendant sa grossesse et donné le jour à un enfant de 3,3 kg. Ces apports valables pour les pays industrialisés où le pourcentage de protéines d'origine animale dans la ration est important sont loin d'être fournis aux femmes enceintes mal nourries de manière chronique dans le tiers-monde. Pour les vitamines et les minéraux, si les besoins sont accrus durant la grossesse, les valeurs exactes ne sont pas connues. Dans les conditions normales les besoins sont couverts à l'exception du fer dont la carence est la plus fréquente même dans des populations autrement bien nourries. Il faut aussi ajouter les problèmes liés à la carence en iode qui frappe des régions entières du globe.

— *Les effets de l'anesthésie et de l'utilisation de divers médicaments sur le nouveau né.* L'importance fondamentale dès la naissance du contact mère-enfant sur la mise en route de l'allaitement maternel demande la plus grande prudence dans l'utilisation durant le travail de drogues qui pourraient gêner ce processus. Barbituriques, analgésiques, tranquillisants passent facilement la barrière placentaire et affectent le système nerveux central. De même le contact visuel mère-enfant ne devrait pas être retardé par les instillations de gouttes oculaires. Cette pratique abandonnée dans certains pays devrait tout au moins être retardée.

— *L'importance du contact mère-enfant immédiatement après la naissance.* L'importance de la période du post-partum pour le développement de l'enfant a été vérifiée. C'est une phase critique qui imprime une marque définitive aux liens psycho-affectifs qui unissent la mère à son enfant. Les interactions multiples qui s'établissent à ce stade sont déterminantes pour l'initiation de la lactation même si un certain septicisme se fait jour sur les effets à long terme de cette relation.

References

1. **Durnin, J.V.G.A.** Energy requirements of pregnancy—an integrated study in five countries: background and methods. *Lancet,* **2**: 895–896 (1987).
2. **Whitehead, R.G. et al.** Incremental dietary needs to support pregnancy. In: *Proceedings of the XIII International Congress of Nutrition.* London, J. Libbey, 1985, pp. 599–603.
3. WHO Technical Report Series No. 724, 1985 (*Energy and protein requirements*: report of a Joint FAO/WHO/UNU Expert Consultation).
4. **Department of Health and Social Security.** *Recommended daily amounts of food energy and nutrients for groups of people in the United Kingdom.* (Rep. Health Soc. Subjects, No. 15), London, HMSO, 1979.
5. **Tuazon, M.A.G. et al.** Energy requirements of pregnancy in the Philippines. *Lancet,* **2**: 1129–1130 (1987).
6. **Joop, M.A. et al.** Body fat mass and basal metabolic rate in Dutch women before, during and after pregnancy: a reappraisal of energy cost during pregnancy. *Am. j. clin. nutr.,* **49**: 765–772 (1989).
7. **DeMaeyer, E. & Adiels-Tegman, M.** The prevalence

of anaemia in the world. *World health statistics quarterly*, **38**: 302–316 (1985).

8. *Requirements of vitamin A, iron, folate and vitamin B_{12}: report of a Joint FAO/WHO Expert Consultation.* Rome, Food and Agriculture Organization, 1988.

9. **Hetzel, B.S. et al.**, ed. *The prevention and control of iodine-deficiency disorders.* Amsterdam, Elsevier, 1987.

10. **Kübler, W.** [Nutrition during pregnancy.] *Der Gynäkolog*, **20**: 83–87 (1987) (in German).

11. **Ledermann, S.A.** Physiological changes of pregnancy and their relation to nutrient needs. In: *Feeding the mother and infant.* New York, Wiley & Sons, 1985.

12. **Naismith, D.J.** Endocrine factors in the control of nutrient utilization in pregnancy. In: Aebi, J. & Whitehead, R., ed. *Maternal nutrition during pregnancy and lactation.* Bern, Huber, 1980.

13. **Naismith, D.J.** Diet during pregnancy—a rationale for prescription. In: Dobbing, J., ed. *Maternal nutrition in pregnancy—eating for two?* London, Academic Press, 1981.

14. **Schneider, H.** [Pregnancy and nutrition.] *Geburtsh. u. Frauenheilk.*, **45**: 135–139 (1985) (in German).

15. **Widdowson, E.M.** The demands of the fetal and maternal tissues for nutrients, and the bearing of these on the needs of the mother to "eat for two". In: Dobbing, J., ed. *Maternal nutrition in pregnancy—eating for two?* London, Academic Press, 1981, pp. 1–17.

16. **Hill, E.P. & Longo, L.D.** Dynamics of maternal–fetal nutrient transfer. *Federation proceedings*, **39**: 239–244 (1980).

17. **Hauguel, S. & Girard, J.** The role of the placenta in fetal nutrition. In: *Proceedings of the XIII International Congress of Nutrition.* London, J. Libbey, 1985, pp. 604–607.

18. **Battaglia, F.G. & Meschia, G.** Principal substrates of fetal metabolism. *Physiol. rev.*, **58**: 499–527 (1978).

19. **Hay, W.W. et al.** Fetal glucose uptake and utilization as functions of maternal glucose concentration. *Am. j. physiol.*, **246**: E237–242 (1984).

20. **Young, M.** Placental factors and fetal nutrition. *Am. j. clin. nutr.*, **34** (Suppl. 4): 738–743 (1981).

21. **Kalkhoff, R.K. et al.** Carbohydrate and lipid metabolism during normal pregnancy: relationship to gestational hormone action. *Semin. perinat.*, **4**: 291–307 (1978).

22. **Van Lierde, M. et al.** Ultrasonic measurement of aortic and umbilical blood flow in the human fetus. *Obstet. gynec.*, **63**: 801–805 (1984).

23. **Meschia, G.** Circulation to female reproductive organs. In: *Handbook of physiology, the cardiovascular system III.* Bethesda, The American Physiological Society, 1984.

24. **Ruzycki, S.M. et al.** Placental amino acid uptake. IV. Transport by microvillous membrane vesicles. *Am. j. physiol.*, **234**: C27–C35 (1978).

25. **Grünberger, W. et al.** [Hypotension in pregnancy and fetal outcome.] *Fortschr. Med.*, **97** (4): 141–144 (1979) (in German, English abstract).

26. **Munro, H.N. et al.** The placenta in nutrition. *Ann. rev. nutr.*, **3**: 97–124 (1983).

27. **Posner, B.I.** Insulin receptors in human and animal placental tissue. *Diabetes*, **23**: 209–217 (1974).

28. **Zimmermann, T. et al.** Oxidation and synthesis of fatty acids in human and rat placental and fetal tissues. *Biol. neonate*, **36**: 109 (1981).

29. **Carroll, M.J. & Young, M.** The relationship between placental protein synthesis and transfer of amino acids. *Biochem. j.*, **210**: 99–105 (1983).

30. **Barness, L.A.** Nutrition for healthy neonates. In: Gracey, M. & Falkner, F.F., ed. *Nutritional needs and assessment of normal growth.* New York, Raven Press, 1985.

31. *Minor and trace elements in breast milk. Report of a Joint WHO/IAEA Collaborative Study.* Geneva, World Health Organization, 1989.

32. WHO Technical Report Series No. 532, 1973 (*Trace elements in human nutrition*: report of a WHO Expert Committee).

33. **American Academy of Pediatrics, Committee on Nutrition.** Water requirements in relation to osmolar load as it applies to infant feeding. *Pediatrics*, **19**: 338–343 (1957).

34. **Almroth, S.** Water requirements of breast-fed infants in a hot climate. *Am. j. clin. nutr.*, **31**: 1154–1157 (1978).

35. **Goldberg, N.M. & Adams, E.** Supplementary water for breast-fed babies in a hot and dry climate—not really a necessity. *Arch. dis. child.*, **58**: 73–74 (1983).

36. **Auerbach, K.G. & Gartner, L.M.** Breast-feeding and human milk: their association with jaundice in the neonate. *Clin. perinatol.*, **14**: 89–107 (1987).

37. **MacLaurin, J.C.** Changes in body water distribution during the first two weeks of life. *Arch. dis. child*, **41**: 286–291 (1966).

38. **Hansen, J.D.L. & Smith, C.A.** Effects of withholding fluid in the immediate postnatal period. *Pediatrics*, **12**: 99–113 (1953).

39. **Coulter, D.M. & Avery, M.E.** Paradoxical reduction in tissue hydration with weight gain in neonatal rabbit pups. *Ped. res.*, **14**: 1122–1126 (1980).

40. **Lorenz, K. & Bingerben, N.** The normal parent–newborn relationship. In: Marx, G.F., ed. *Clinical management of mother and newborn.* New York, Springer, 1979.

41. **Hersher, L. et al.** Modifiability of the critical period for the development of maternal behaviour in sheep and goats. *Int. j. comp. ethol.*, **20**: 311–320 (1974).

42. **Klaus, M. et al.** Maternal attachment—importance of the first postpartum days. *New Engl. j. med.*, **286**: 460–462 (1972).

43. **Klaus, M. & Kennell, J.** *Maternal infant bonding, the effect of early separation and loss on family development.* St. Louis, Mosby, 1976.

44. **Hales, D.J. et al.** Defining the limits of the maternal sensitive period. *Develop. med. child. neurol.*, **19** (4): 454–461 (1977).

45. **DeChateau, P.** The first hour after delivery—its impact on synchrony of the parent–infant relationship. *Pediatrician*, **9**: 151–168 (1980).

46. **Bowen, S.M. & Miller, B.C.** Paternal attachment behaviour. *Nursing res.*, **5**: 307–311 (1980).

47. **Cobliner, W.G.** The normal parent–newborn relation-

ship. Its importance for the healthy development of the child. In: Marx, G.F., ed. *Clinical management of mother and newborn*. New York, Springer, 1979.

48. **Leboyer, F.** *Pour une naissance sans violence*. Paris, Seuil, 1974.

49. **Klaus, M.H. et al.** Human maternal behaviour at the first contact with her young. *Pediatrics*, **46**: 187–192 (1970).

50. **Sosa, R. et al.** The effect of early mother–infant contact on breast-feeding, infection and growth. In: *Breast-feeding and the mother*. Amsterdam, Elsevier, 1976 (Ciba Foundation Symposium 45 (new series)), pp. 179–193.

51. Maternal attachment and mother–neonate bonding: a critical review. In: Lamb, M.E. & Brown, A.L., ed. *Advances in developmental psychology. Vol. 2*. Hillsdale, NJ, Lawrence Erlbaum Ass., 1982.

52. **Matthews, M.K.**, The relationship between maternal labour, analgesia and delay in the initiation of breastfeeding in healthy neonates in the early neonatal period. *Midwifery*, **5**: 3–10 (1989).

53. **Brazelton, T.B.** Effect of maternal medication on the neonate and his behavior. *J. pediatr.* **58**: 513–554 (1961).

54. **Kron, R. et al.** Newborn sucking behavior affected by obstetric sedation. *Pediatrics*, **37**: 1012–1016 (1966).

55. **Hodgkinson, R.** Effects of obstetric analgesia—anaesthesia on neonatal neurobehaviour. In: Marx, G.F., ed. *Clinical management of mother and newborn*. New York, Springer, 1979.

56. **Borgstedt, A.D. & Rosen, M.G.** Medication during labor correlated with behavior and EEG of the newborn. *Am. j. dis. child.*, **115**: 21–24 (1968).

57. **Hughes, J.G. et al.** Electroencephalography of the newborn. I. Brain potentials of babies born of mothers given meperidine hydrochloride, vinbarbital

sodium or morphine. *Am. j. dis. child.*, **79**: 996–1007 (1950).

58. **Hughes, J.G. et al.** Electroencephalography of the newborn. III. Brain potentials of the babies born of mothers given seconal sodium. *Am. j. dis. child.*, **76**: 626–633 (1948).

59. **Fraser, C.M.** Routine perinatal procedures, their necessity and psychosocial effects. *Acta obst. gyn. Scand.*, Suppl. 117: 1–39 (1983).

60. *Having a baby in Europe*: report on a study. Copenhagen, WHO Regional Office for Europe, 1985 (Public Health in Europe No. 26).

61. **Gesell, A.L. & Ilg, F.** *Feeding behaviour of infants. A pediatric approach to the mental hygiene of early life*. Philadelphia, J.B. Lippincott, 1937.

62. **Hellbrügge, T. et al.** Circadian periodicity of physiologic functions in different stages of infancy and childhood. *Ann. N.Y. Acad. Sci.*, **117**: 361–373 (1964).

63. Guidelines in infant nutrition. III. Recommendations for infant feeding. European Society for Paediatrics, Gastroenterology and Nutrition (ESPGAN) Committee on Nutrition. *Acta paed. Scand.*, Suppl. No. 302 (1982).

64. **Herrera, M.G. et al.**, ed. Maternal weight/height and the effect of food supplementation during pregnancy and lactation. In: Aebi, H. & Whitehead, R., ed. *Maternal nutrition during pregnancy and lactation: a Nestlé Foundation workshop*. Bern, Hans Huber, 1980, pp. 252–263.

65. **Lechtig, A. & Klein, R.E.** Maternal food supplementation and infant health: results of a study in rural areas of Guatemala. In: Aebi, H. & Whitehead, R., ed. *Maternal nutrition during pregnancy and lactation: a Nestlé Foundation workshop*. Bern, Hans Huber, 1980, pp. 285–313.

2. Lactation

Lactation is the most energy-efficient way to provide for the dietary needs of young mammals, their mother's milk being actively protective, immunomodulatory, and ideal for their needs. Intrauterine mammary gland development in the human female is already apparent by the end of the sixth week of gestation. During puberty and adolescence secretions of the anterior pituitary stimulate the maturation of the graafian follicles In the ovaries and stimulate the secretion of follicular estrogens, which stimulate development of the mammary ducts. Pregnancy has the most dramatic effect on the breast, but development of the glandular breast tissue and deposition of fat and connective tissue continue under the influence of cyclic sex-hormone stimulation. Many changes occur in the nipple and breast during pregnancy and at delivery as a prelude to lactation. Preparation of the breasts is so effective that lactation could commence even if pregnancy were discontinued at 16 weeks.

Following birth, placental inhibition of milk synthesis is removed, and a woman's progesterone blood levels decline rapidly. The breasts fill with milk, which is a high-density, low-volume feed called colostrum until about 30 hours after birth. Because it is not the level of maternal hormones, but the efficiency of infant suckling and/or milk removal that governs the volume of milk produced in each breast, mothers who permit their infants to feed ad libitum commonly observe that they have large volumes of milk 24–48 hours after birth. The two maternal reflexes involved in lactation are the milk-production and milk-ejection reflex. A number of complementary reflexes are involved when the infant feeds: the rooting reflex (which programmes the infant to search for the nipple), the sucking reflex (rhythmic jaw action creating negative pressure and a peristaltic action of the tongue), and the swallowing reflex. The infant's instinctive actions need to be consolidated into learned behaviour in the postpartum period when the use of artificial teats and dummies (pacifiers) may condition the infant to different oral actions that are inappropriate for breast-feeding.

Comparisons of breast milk and cow's milk fail to describe the many important differences between them, e.g., the structural and qualitative differences in proteins and fats, and the bioavailability of minerals. The protection against infection and allergies conferred on the infant, which is impossible to attain through any other feeding regimen, is one of breast milk's most outstanding qualities. The maximum birth-spacing effect of lactation is achieved when an infant is fully, or nearly fully, breast-fed and the mother consequently remains amenorrhoeic.

Introduction

Lactation is a characteristic of mammals alone, and this ability to provide an ideal food for their young, regardless of the season, confers an evolutionary advantage over other species. Even where food is plentiful, lactation is the most energy-efficient way to provide for the dietary needs of the young. In situations of scarcity, the ability of mammals to efficiently utilize low-quality food resources in order to keep the female alive, to provide high-quality nutrition for the infant, and to regulate births is crucial to the survival of both mother and offspring. This is true in humans no less than in other mammals; as an important survival mechanism, mammals have developed many strategies both to optimize lactation's contribution to the development of the young and to reduce the metabolic burden thereby imposed on the female.

Human lactation is a relatively neglected area of scientific research. In fact, less is known about lactation in humans than in commercially exploited animals, and many of the beliefs and practices that sometimes prevent successful lactation in humans have no parallel in animal husbandry. Because there are still so many unanswered questions about the physiology of human lactation, this chapter will require regular up-dating as it is unable to cover many clinically relevant issues.

Development of the female breast

During intrauterine growth and childhood

Intrauterine mammary gland development is apparent by the end of the sixth week of gestation with the appearance of an ectodermal ridge consisting of 4–6 layers of cells at the site of the glands. These layers gradually thicken and invade the underlying mesenchymal tissue in the following weeks, while the smooth muscle of the areola and nipple develops simultaneously.

At about fifteen weeks, the cells invading the mesenchyme bud into 15–25 epithelial strips, which later become the breast segments. Vascularization and formation of specific apocrine glands (Montgomery glands) occur at the same time. By eight months, canalization is complete and differentiation into alveolar structures takes place, accompanied by increased vascularization and formation of fat and connective tissue. The mammary connective tissue serves as a carrier of blood vessels and supports the smooth musculature of the areola and nipple. The inner layers surround the mammary ducts and support glandular elements.

The early stages of intrauterine mammary development are independent of any specific hormonal effects. Only the main lactiferous ducts are present at birth. Despite this, the placental sex hormones, which entered the fetal circulation in the last stages of pregnancy, may stimulate the neonatal breast to secrete milk ("witch's milk") at 2–3 days postpartum. This secretion subsides spontaneously in the next days or weeks, and should be ignored; manipulation of the infant's breasts can lead to mastitis. Neonatal breast development then regresses into the small mammary disk of childhood and remains at rest for the most part until pre-puberty (1).

During puberty and adolescence

With the onset of hypothalamic maturation in the female at 10–12 years of age, the secretion of gonadotrophins (FSH, LH) from the anterior pituitary stimulates the maturation of the graafian follicles in the ovaries and initiates the secretion of follicular estrogens, which stimulate development of the mammary ducts. The volume and elasticity of the connective tissues surrounding the ducts increase, and vascularization and fat deposition are enhanced. These developments become obvious as an enlargement of the breast disc at about twelve years of age. Thus, estrogens are mainly responsible for breast development for the first 2–3 years after the onset of puberty. The complete development of the breasts into their adolescent size and structure requires the combined effects of estrogens and progesterone, as does the pigmentation of the areola. Although the differentiation of the breast tissue takes place during adolescence, changes in the breast continue throughout a woman's life. Pregnancy has the most dramatic effect on the breast (see below), but development of the glandular breast tissue, and deposition of fat and connective tissue continue under the influence of cyclic sex-hormone stimulation.

Anatomy and morphology of the mature breast

In the mature woman the breast contains perhaps 15–25 segments or lobes of glandular tissue, surrounded by connective tissue. Not every lobe is functional in each lactation, or for the duration of any lactation; particular lobes may regress sooner than others. Women can successfully feed a singleton infant with only one functional breast (2), or with only parts of both breasts fully functional. This is well documented after surgery of many kinds, including reduction mammoplasty, breast biopsy or enlargement. Successfully breast-feeding more than one child requires a greater amount of functional glandular tissue, and the recorded value of milk produced by wet-nurses and mothers of twins or triplets (3) makes it clear that many women never achieve their potential for milk production. With each subsequent lactation, functional glandular tissue generally increases.

The structure of the breast has been likened to a tree with trunk, branches and leaves: the milk ducts form the trunk and branches linked with the tiny, sac-like alveoli, which are the leaves (4). Milk is secreted in the alveoli, of which there are 10–100 clusters in each segment enveloped in collagen sheaths. The sheaths, in turn, prolong the small ducts emptying into the main milk duct. Underneath this collagen sheath is a lining of contractile myoepithelial cells, which surrounds the glandular structure. These cells contract under the influence of oxytocin, assisting milk to flow from the alveoli into the ducts (see below).

The main milk ducts are more distensible in the area just beneath the areola. Some milk collects in what are sometimes referred to as the lactiferous sinuses, which are compressed both during suckling and when milk is expressed by hand. Several milk ducts may merge before they reach the nipple, so that the number of openings in the nipple does not correspond to the number of lobes in the breast.

The nipple is located in the middle of the circular, pigmented areola, which probably serves as a visual marker for the infant. The nipple is usually elevated a few millimetres from the skin surface but its size and shape can vary widely between individuals without any loss of function. The areola contains smooth muscle and collagenous connective tissue fibres in circular and radial arrangements. It is usually 3–5 cm in diameter in adult women, but the range is quite wide. Some women have no visible pigmented area, while on others it may occupy half the breast; both groups lactate successfully.

Both the areola and nipple are heavily innervated. The sensitivity of the nipple-areola complex increases during pregnancy and is greatest in the first few days after birth (5). The nipple (like the cornea) contains unmyelinated nerve endings, and so is extremely painful when traumatized by an inadequately positioned infant (6) (see below). Appropriate stimulation of the nerve endings causes nipple erection and triggers the pituitary reflex mechanisms that release oxytocin and prolactin. The areola also contains structures related to the apocrine Montgomery glands, which probably serve as both lubricating and scent organs during lactation (7).

Changes in the nipple during pregnancy

An increase in nipple sensitivity is one of the first signs of pregnancy in many women. The areola surrounding the nipple may increase in diameter during pregnancy, and the Montgomery tubercles, or glands, increase in prominence and begin secreting a sebaceous substance having anti-bacterial properties. Nipple changes during pregnancy have an effect on the infant's later ability to remove milk efficiently. The nipples enlarge and become more protractile, which has been measured by compressing the areola immediately behind the nipple. The more protractile the nipple and breast tissue behind it, the more easily an infant can breast-feed. It is the protractility of breast tissue (rather than the shape and size of the nipple) that determines whether the nipple can be drawn far enough into the infant's mouth to avoid being traumatized by infant oral activity, and whether the infant has a sufficient mouthful of breast to extract milk efficiently (see below). Infants *breast*-feed; the nipple is the conduit through which milk flows, and probably serves as an oral stimulus to initiate feeding behaviour. Extreme, intractable nipple inversion, which often involves tightness and tethering of breast tissue as well, can make breast-feeding difficult or even impossible (see chapter 3); fortunately, this is rare. It is not unusual, however, for nipple inversion to be mistakenly diagnosed when a normal flat nipple is further effaced during breast engorgement.

Changes in the breast during pregnancy and after delivery

During pregnancy intensive lobular development occurs under the influence of placental lactogen, as well as the luteal and placental sex steroids. Prolactin is increasingly released and contributes to breast development. Ducts and alveoli multiply and develop so rapidly that already at 5–8 weeks in many women the breasts are visibly enlarged and feel heavier, pigmentation of the areola is intensified, and the superficial veins become dilated. However, as glandular development proceeds, fat stores in some women may be mobilized and removed from the breasts, with the result that there is little noticeable change in breast volume, although these women subsequently lactate successfully. After delivery, the volume of each breast grows by an average of about 225 ml (8) due to a doubling of blood flow, increased secretion, and development of glandular tissue, partially filled with colostrum, sometimes from midpregnancy. Colostrum may leak from the breast, depending on such varied factors as ambient temperature and the tone of the sphincter muscles that control spontaneous outflow. In all these developments there is normally wide variation between individuals but none of these factors is predictive of success or failure in breast-feeding.

During the early months of pregnancy, ductular sprouting is pronounced owing to the influence of estrogen. With an increase in progesterone levels after three months, development of the alveoli exceeds duct formation, and the progressive increase in prolactin stimulates glandular activity and the secretion of colostrum, the earliest milk. The point at which the breasts develop the capacity to synthesize milk constituents is referred to as lactogenesis I (9). Larger-volume milk production is inhibited by placental sex steroids, particularly progesterone. This inhibition is so powerful that even small fragments of retained placental material can delay lactogenesis II, or the time when more copious milk secretion begins after birth. The preparation of the breasts for lactation is so effective, however, that lactation could commence even at 16 weeks if pregnancy were discontinued.

Lactation

Onset of lactation

Milk synthesis in the alveoli is a complex process involving four secretory mechanisms: exocytosis, fat synthesis and transfer, secretion of ions and water, and immunoglobulin transfer from the extracellular space. These are of little direct clinical relevance and are reviewed elsewhere (10).

Following birth, placental inhibition of milk synthesis is removed, and a woman's progesterone blood levels decline rapidly. The breasts fill with milk, which is colostrum until about 30 hours after birth. At between 30 and 40 hours (11) there is a rapid change in milk composition as the amount of lactose synthesized increases and milk volume thus rises, lactose being the most osmotically active milk component. This rise in milk volume usually occurs before a woman notices any breast fullness and engorgement or other signs of the uncomfortable subjective experience that is often described as "milk coming in".

Mothers who permit their infants to feed *ad libitum* commonly observe that they have a large volume of milk by 24–48 hours after birth, but experience no engorgement. It is now thought that the event described as "milk coming in" marks the shift from lactation driven by endocrine control to lactation under autocrine control (12), when it is the removal of milk from the breasts, in a continuing favourable hormonal milieu, which governs milk production. Some mothers may experience this transition from endocrine control to autocrine control as a sensation of fullness and increased warmth in the breasts, as the build-up of intramammary pressure accompanying the build-up of suppressor peptides in the glands begins to down-regulate the volume of milk produced to that required by the baby (i.e., equal to the amount that is being removed from the breasts). Increasing fullness occurs when inefficient milk removal, combined with increased blood flow to the breasts, creates lymphatic oedema, which in turn can contribute to limiting the milk outflow, permitting the accumulation of suppressor peptides, and eventually decreasing the milk secretion (see below).

Because lactation is an energy-intensive process, it makes evolutionary sense that there should be inbuilt safeguards against wasteful over-production as well as mechanisms to permit a prompt response to increased infant need. Recent research has confirmed that such mechanisms exist in humans as in other mammals. It is not the level of maternal hormones, but the efficiency of infant suckling and/or milk removal, which governs the volume produced in each breast. Both breasts are subject to the same hormonal influences, but the volume each produces corresponds to that removed by the infant. Many women successfully breast-feed from one breast only; in such cases the unused breast involutes.

Maintenance of lactation

Maternal reflexes. The two maternal reflexes involved in lactation are the *milk-production* and *milk-ejection* reflex. Both involve hormones (prolactin and oxytocin, respectively), and both are responsive to lactation's driving force, which is suckling. Stimulation by the infant of nerve endings in the nipple-areola complex sends impulses through afferent neural-reflex pathways to the hypothalamus, resulting in the secretion of prolactin from the anterior pituitary and oxytocin from the posterior pituitary. Other hormones (cortisol, insulin, thyroid and parathyroid hormones, and growth hormone) also support lactation (13). Prolactin is a key lactogenic hormone, stimulating the initial alveolar production of milk; it induces messenger- and transfer RNA for milk-protein synthesis, and influences alpha-lactalbumin, and hence lactose synthesis, in the alveolar cells. Other functions of prolactin include water and salt conservation through the kidneys and, possibly, prolongation of postpartum amenorrhoea through its effect on the ovaries; both these functions reduce the metabolic stress of lactation.

As distinct from its role in initiating lactation, the importance of prolactin in sustaining lactation is the subject of considerable scientific debate (14). Serum prolactin levels in non-pregnant women are about 10 ng/ml; its concentration gradually increases during pregnancy but decreases sharply after delivery. At four weeks postpartum the mean is about 20–30 ng/ml in lactating women, and 10 ng/ml in non-lactating women. However, the basal serum level of prolactin, at which satisfactory milk production is reached and can be sustained, varies widely between women after the early postpartum period (15). Some women lactate successfully with basal prolactin levels equivalent to those of non-lactating women. In early lactation suckling induces a surge of prolactin to about ten times the basal pre-suckling levels after about 20–30 minutes. By three months this response is markedly decreased, and by six months it has virtually disappeared in most women. Yet suckling and the removal of milk allow milk production to be sustained on a supply and demand basis, catering to the infant's needs. For reasons not yet understood, maternal malnutrition is associated with considerable elevation of basal prolactin levels (16).

As well as inducing the release of prolactin from the anterior pituitary, the infant's feeding also excites cholinergic fibres in the hypothalamus and stimulates the release of oxytocin from the posterior pituitary. Oxytocin has a short half-life and is secreted predominantly in short pulses. Since it is very difficult to assay (17), little is known about the levels of oxytocin in pregnant, non-pregnant, and lactating women. However, it is estimated that about 100 mU oxytocin are released in ten minutes of breast-feeding (18). It is not known whether this is affected by the large doses of oxytocin that are used to augment labour. Oxytocin contracts the myoepithelial cells, forcing the milk out into the ducts. The force of the contractions can initially be very strong and painful for some women, and the milk can be ejected many centimetres from the breast; more usually it simply drips from one breast as the infant drinks from the other.

Mothers may experience this milk-ejection reflex, or milk "let-down", as a warm and tingling sensation in the breast, or as a feeling of pressure, or they may not notice it at all unless they watch the baby's feeding rhythm. Intramammary pressure does rise, and increased blood flow is obvious with thermography. Contractions in the uterus are also induced; this assists speedy and complete uterine involution, but can be extremely painful, particularly for multigravid mothers, for some days after delivery (19). These women may need explanation and reassurance and, in severe cases, some form of pain relief.

The importance of oxytocin to milk release varies according to the mammalian species. Traditional dairy animals have large lactiferous sinuses, or cisterns, which allow for up to 50% of milk to be obtained independently of the milk-ejection reflex. In species not so equipped—including rats, rabbits, pigs, dogs and humans—very little milk can be obtained in the absence of the milk-ejection reflex. However, serious defects in this reflex are clinically rare. It seems to be most sensitive to disturbance during the early neonatal period, which underlines the importance of allowing women to breast-feed under conditions that they find comfortable.

The milk-ejection reflex responds not only to tactile stimuli but can be triggered by visual, olfactory, or auditory (20) stimuli (particularly in the early days of lactation); it can also be conditioned (21). Physical closeness to, or thinking about, an infant can trigger milk ejection in some women through a contraction of the myoepithelial cells. This can occur in some women years after lactation has ceased, even though ejection is not possible in the absence of milk. Conversely, this reflex can be temporarily inhibited by the effects of adrenalin (22), e.g., in some women subject to sudden, extremely unpleasant, or painful physical or psychological stimuli.

Minor or chronic stress has not been shown to affect the milk-ejection reflex other than to delay it slightly. Some women do experience a genuine inability to release milk even when their breasts are obviously full. The most usual explanation for this is not psychological but physical; owing to limited suckling their breasts are overfull, and the resulting extreme back-pressure prevents oxytocin from contracting the myoepithelial cells. Warmth, pumping, or skilful hand-expression of some milk can decrease this pressure and enable the reflex to operate. Temporary inhibition, or simple delay in milk ejection, is relatively common. It can be readily overcome by cajoling the infant to persevere for the minute it may take for the suckling stimulus to operate. Unfortunately, in cases where women are subjected to negative messages about their capacity to lactate, this temporary inhibition of milk ejection is frequently misinterpreted as a sign of "milk insufficiency"; the introduction of supplementary feeds only contributes to making the feared insufficiency a reality (see chapter 3).

The responsiveness of the milk-ejection reflex explains why successful breast-feeding has been described as a "confidence trick". If a mother truly believes that she can provide milk for her infant, she will encounter few problems with milk let-down, even in the stressful conditions and overwork experienced by most of the world's lactating women. Research from the Gambia confirms this (2). If, on the other hand, a woman believes that modern life is incompatible with full breast-feeding, she may be more

inclined to interpret any difficulties encountered—ironically, even those arising from producing too great a volume—as being due to too little milk. Women need basic information about the mechanics of breast-feeding and the reliability of lactation; as a survival mechanism it is not easily disturbed except by powerful physiological forces, or interference with its basic mechanism, appropriate suckling.

Nineteenth century ignorance of these basic physiological facts and of the adverse conditions under which lactation proceeds uneventfully the world over accounts for this same era's traditional insistence that "the secretion of milk proceeds best in a tranquil state of mind and a cheerful manner" (23). Relaxed interaction with one's infant is no doubt preferable for a host of reasons, but it is also a luxury that is unavailable to many women. Even the original sudden painful experiments used to demonstrate inhibition of milk ejection under stress showed that the effect was short-lived (24) and reduced, rather than prevented, milk transfer.

Both oxytocin and prolactin affect a mother's mood and physical state, and the latter hormone is considered crucial to appropriate maternal behaviour in various species. The effects of bromocriptine or other prolactin-antagonists on mother–infant interaction have not been studied. New research about oxytocin (25) suggests that it, too, is a "bonding" hormone, with important consequences for relationships between both sexual partners and mother and child. Recent studies have begun to explore how the chosen feeding method affects a mother's subsequent adjustment to her infant (26).

Infant reflexes. The normal full-term human infant at birth is equipped to breast-feed successfully. Like other mammalian newborns, left to their own devices human infants will follow an innate programme of pre-feeding behaviour in the first hours after birth that can include crawling from the mother's abdomen to her breast, coordinated hand-mouth activity, active searching for the nipple while the mouth gapes widely, and finally, attaching well to the breast and feeding vigorously before falling asleep—all this within 120–150 minutes after delivery (27). The key to lactation maintenance is appropriate infant-feeding behaviour, which means emptying the breasts efficiently, frequently, and for long-enough periods both to maintain lactogenic hormonal levels and to prevent the build-up in the breasts of compounds that suppress lactation (see below).

A number of complementary reflexes are involved when the infant feeds. The *rooting reflex* programmes the infant to search for the nipple while gaping widely enough to take in a good mouthful of breast tissue. When the infant's cheek or mouth is touched, the infant gapes and turns towards the stimulus, attempting to grasp it orally. The *sucking reflex* is triggered when something touches the palate. In fact, "sucking" is something of a misnomer for this action, which consists of rhythmic jaw action creating negative pressure, and a peristaltic action of the tongue, which strips milk from the breast and moves it to the throat, where it triggers the swallowing reflex. This feeding action also stimulates the synthesis and secretion of lactogenic hormones that evoke the mother's milk-production and ejection reflexes, and removes the peptides that might suppress alveolar milk synthesis. Recent ultrasound studies have provided excellent illustrations (28) of this process of breast-feeding; it differs markedly both from previous verbal descriptions of how infants breast-feed and from printed descriptions of how infants feed from artificial teats.

In the normal neonate, breast-feeding reflexes are already strong at birth. Indeed, evidence now confirms that some infants as young as 32 weeks gestation and as small as 1200 g are capable of breast-feeding efficiently even before they can feed from artificial teats, which are associated with hypoxia and bradycardia in premature infants (29). However, these crucial reflexes may be weak or absent in extremely pre-term or very-low-birthweight (see chapter 5) or sick infants. Cerebral damage, congenital defects, generalized infection (septicaemia), and severe jaundice may also cause feeding difficulties. Physical defects such as cleft lip or palate (see chapter 3) pose individual challenges, depending on the interaction between the defect and the mother's breast. However, the most common causes of decreased efficiency of these reflexes are in fact iatrogenic: obstetrical sedation or analgesia (see chapters 1 and 3), and interference in the process of learning in the period after birth. The infant's instinctive actions need to be consolidated into learned behaviour in the postpartum period. The use of other oral objects, whether teats or dummies (pacifiers), in the neonatal period may condition the infant to different oral actions that are inappropriate for breast-feeding.

In the early postpartum period, lactational reflexes are particularly responsive to changes in suckling frequency, duration and adequacy. To *initiate* breast-feeding successfully, infants should be allowed to breast-feed within an hour of birth, when both their reflexes and their mother's sensitivity to tactile stimuli of the areola and nipple are strongest. To *establish* breast-feeding successfully, factors that decrease the duration, efficiency and frequency of infant suckling should be eliminated as far as possible

(30). These factors include limitation of feeding time, scheduled feeds, poor positioning, the use of other oral objects, and giving the infant other fluids, e.g., water, sugar solutions, and vegetable- or animal-milk products. The giving of formula milk not only decreases an infant's appetite for breast milk, but also increases the risk of infection and allergy (31). Ideally, mothers and babies should be left in close skin contact after an uncomplicated delivery without use of drugs; recent Swedish studies have shown that separation from the mother and analgesia during labour (32) were the factors most closely associated with suckling difficulty. Following this early contact, mothers should be encouraged to feed their infants as often and as long as needed. Excessively long feeds or the development of nipple trauma indicate that help is required (33, 34). The use of creams, lotions, sprays or other applications for sore nipples has little proven basis and may in fact only create additional problems, which increase the risk of further trauma (35) (see Annex 1).

Cessation of lactation

Milk secretion continues for some time after the cessation of suckling. In normal circumstances, lactation will continue in each breast for as long as milk is being removed from it. As the volume of milk decreases, its composition changes; higher levels of fat, sodium and immunoglobulins, and lower levels of lactose are usual (36). Although most mammals "dry up" within 5 days of the last suckling episode, the period of involution in women averages 40 days. Within this period it is relatively easy to re-establish full lactation if the infant resumes frequent suckling. In many societies weaning children do revert to full breast-feeding when challenged by disease, and thus a process of gradual involution has obvious advantages for the infant; it also has advantages for the mother. In abrupt weaning, it takes two days for immunoglobulin and lactoferrin levels to rise, which leaves the breast vulnerable to infection. This is undoubtedly part of the reason for higher rates of abscess formation in women with mastitis who stop feeding from the affected breast (see chapter 3).

As discussed earlier, after the initial period the breasts are under autocrine control; it is the build-up in the glandular tissue of inhibiting peptides that brings about the cessation of milk secretion. This makes the management of early lactation, and of mastitis, particularly important. Whenever unphysiological feeding practices prevent the efficient removal of milk, secretion will decrease. Virtually all women initially produce more milk than their infants can consume. The breasts should not be permitted to become over-full, tight and lumpy at any time during the first week. Women should be shown how to check their breasts for lumpiness (particularly in the axilla and around breast margins); to recognize obstruction of outflow building up in the breast; and to relieve this by gentle hand expression or other means. Otherwise whole lobes of breast tissue may stop secretion, as they will when outflow is impeded by permanent damage such as scar tissue from burns or reconstructive surgery. (In most surgical patients a carefully supervised trial of lactation is advised, as many functional lobes may retain outlets that permit full or partial lactation.) Fortunately, in the normal postpartum woman, the decrease in secretion is likely to be temporary if the infant continues to suckle, and the mother does not supplement with artificial feeds. The milk output seems to be most sensitive in the first weeks to the suckling stimulus and the amount of milk removed, although at all stages of lactation increased suckling frequency will result in increased milk supply, usually after about 48 hours (37).

Breast-milk composition

Breast milk and its precursor, colostrum, ensure the neonate's adaptation and successful transition to independent postnatal life. Colostrum is a sticky yellowish fluid which fills the alveolar cells during the last trimester of pregnancy, and is secreted for some days after birth (38). Even where a mother has been feeding an older child throughout pregnancy, her milk will go through a colostral phase just before and after the new birth. The amounts of colostrum secreted vary widely, ranging from 10 to 100 ml/day, with a mean of about 30 ml. This secretion gradually increases and achieves the composition of mature milk by 30–40 hours after birth.

Colostrum is a high-density, low-volume feed. It contains less lactose, fat and water-soluble vitamins than mature milk, but more protein, fat-soluble vitamins (including vitamins E, A, and K) and more of some minerals such as sodium and zinc. It is so high in immunoglobulins and a host of other protective factors that it could be described as nature's prescription as well as nature's food. Colostrum is well-matched to the specific needs of the neonate; immature infant kidneys cannot handle large volumes of fluid without metabolic stress; the production of lactase and other gut enzymes is just beginning; anti-oxidants and quinones are needed for protection against oxidative damage and haemorrhagic disease; immunoglobulins coat the immature gut lining of the infant, preventing adherence of bacterial, viral, parasitic and other pathogens; and growth factors stimulate the infant's own systems in ways science is just beginning to understand. Colostrum, like the milk to come after it, acts as a

modulator of infant development. To dilute its effects by giving water, or negate them by adding other foreign substances to the infant's gastrointestinal tract, is not easily justified.

Colostrum evolves into mature milk between 3 and 14 days postpartum. Mature breast milk has hundreds of recognized components. It is variable in composition not only between mothers, but also in the same mother between breasts, between feeds, and even during a single feed, as well as over the course of lactation. These variations are not considered random but functional, while the infant's role in determining milk variability is increasingly seen as important. Human milk has the potential to meet an infant's individual needs as does the milk of other mammalian species (e.g., the red kangaroo, which provides two quite different milks for different teats for young of different ages). Women feeding twins who have a consistent breast preference sometimes find that their breasts are producing individually tailored milks. As lactation winds down and the breasts involute, regression milk resembles colostrum in its high level of immunoglobulins, which protect both the weanling and the breast itself.

Comparisons of the composition of breast milk and cow's milk, as well as some usual western breast-milk substitutes, are widely available. While they list some of the hundreds of components in milks, they fail to describe the many differences between them. For example, bovine-milk proteins, whether whey or casein, are structurally and qualitatively different from human-milk proteins, and may generate antigenic responses. Bovine lactoferrin may act quite differently in the human infant than it does in the calf; differences in the external carbohydrate structure of the protein may mean that infant receptors for human lactoferrin cannot lock onto, and release, the minerals taken up by bovine lactoferrin. The relative bioavailability of trace minerals (see below) is not obvious from a mere quantitative listing, nor are the qualitative differences between the saturated fats of human milk and atherogenic saturated vegetable fats such as coconut oil (39) obvious from tables listing fats by category. Mammalian milks are all fluids of great complexity, uniquely suited to the needs of the young of the species concerned.

Protein

Mature human milk has the lowest protein concentration among mammals. Based on findings from the WHO study concerning the quantity and quality of breast milk (40), average protein content is accepted as being 1.15 g/100 ml, except during the first month when it is 1.3 g/100 ml, calculated on the basis of total nitrogen × 6.25 (41). There are wide variations between mothers, however, as in the case of ten mothers whose total protein content on the eighth day postpartum was found to range from 1.13 to 2.07 g/100 ml (42). Such differences in milk composition may help explain the equally wide variation in milk intakes observed in thriving breast-fed infants, who are permitted to self-regulate their intake. Some studies have shown that the actual protein content of human milk, when determined on the basis of amino acids, is about 0.8–0.9 g/100 ml (43); non-protein nitrogen (mostly urea (44)) accounted for the other 25–30% of total nitrogen. Nutritionally available protein may be even less than 0.8 g/100 ml when a correction is made for those whey proteins (the anti-infective proteins such as secretory IgA, lysozymes and lactoferrin) that resist proteolysis and are therefore not absorbed. These low breast-milk protein levels are nevertheless more than adequate for optimal growth in young infants, and result in an appropriately low solute load for the infant's immature kidneys.

In the light of this new information, it is now considered that the total protein content of breast-milk substitutes should be lowered even further. Infants fed artificially, whether on the latest whey- or casein-dominant formulas, have elevated blood urea and amino acid levels, and thus higher renal solute loads (45); neither the short- nor long-term metabolic consequences of this finding are known. The high protein and salt content (and consequent renal solute load) of breast-milk substitutes until the 1970s was linked to hypernatraemic dehydration (46). While most infants appear to be remarkably capable of adapting in the short term to this unphysiological metabolic stress, little research has been done on its possible relation to adult circulatory or renal disease (see chapter 4).

The whey:casein ratio of human milk is roughly 80:20, that of bovine milk 20:80, while that of breast-milk substitutes varies from 18:82 to 60:40. It is not clear, however, that modifying the bovine protein ratios to the same as human protein will result in improved absorption and serum amino-acid levels that are closer to those of the breast-fed infant (47). Some studies have shown that casein-dominant breast-milk substitutes achieve a more physiological plasma profile than whey-dominant substitutes (47). Although there are similarities, no bovine-milk protein is identical to any human-milk protein; indeed, they are quite different. The human whey proteins consist mainly of human alpha-lactalbumin, an important component of the enzyme system in lactose synthesis. The dominant bovine whey protein, bovine beta-lactoglobulin, has no human-milk protein counterpart, although it is capable of con-

taminating the milk of women who themselves drink cow's milk, and provoking antigenic responses in atopic infants (48). Human milk's high whey:casein ratio results in the formation of a softer gastric curd, which reduces gastric emptying time (49) and facilitates digestion.

Human milk has higher levels of the free amino acids and cystine, and lower levels of methionine, than does cow's milk. Human milk's cystine: methionine ratio is 2:1, which is almost unique for animal tissues and resembles that of plant tissues (40). Cystine is essential for the fetus and pre-term infant because the enzyme cystathionase, which catalyses the transulfuration of methionine to cystine, is lacking in the brain and liver (50). The level of another amino acid, taurine, is also high in human milk. Taurine is necessary for the conjugation of bile salts (and hence fat absorption) (51), in addition to having a role as a neurotransmitter and neuromodulator in the development of the central nervous system. Because infants, unlike adults, are unable to synthesize taurine from cystine and methionine, it has been suggested that taurine should be conditionally considered an essential amino acid for young children (52). Breast milk meets this need; taurine has been added to some breast-milk substitutes since 1984. There are many other differences in milk protein quantity and quality, which have been reviewed elsewhere (53).

Fat

With few exceptions, the fat content of mature human milk is ideally suited to the human infant, and it evokes a unique physiological response (54). Fat concentrations increase from about 2.0 g/100 ml in colostrum to the mature level of a mean of 4–4.5 g/100 ml at fifteen days postpartum; they remain relatively stable thereafter, although there are considerable inter-individual variations both in total fat content and fatty acid composition (55). Fat is the most variable of milk constituents (56). Circadian fluctuations in fat concentrations occur, with highest concentrations usually recorded in the late morning and early afternoon (57). Variations also occur within feeds; in some women fat concentration in hindmilk is 4–5 times greater than in foremilk. The increased fat in hindmilk was believed to act as a satiety regulator, although this could not be demonstrated when infants were bottle-fed milks of varying fat content (58). However, because later stages of a feed, when milk volume is lower, may be providing a considerable proportion of an infant's total caloric intake for that feed, there should be no arbitrary time limit on any feed (59). Infants are capable of regulating their energy intake by mechanisms not yet understood. Because hindmilk provides a higher energy intake, it is important that a mother who is expressing milk should not simply collect foremilk such as "drip milk" (that collects spontaneously in breast shells worn for the purpose). Such milk would be of inadequate caloric value and particularly unsuitable for preterm infants unless enriched with fat from other batches of human milk (60).

Human-milk fat is secreted in microscopic globules that are smaller than those in cow's milk. Triglycerides dominate, with 98% of the lipids enclosed in the globules. The globular membranes are composed of phospholipids, sterols (especially cholesterol) and proteins. The fatty-acid composition of human milk is relatively stable, consisting of about 42% saturated, and about 57% unsaturated, fatty acids (61). Although the concentrations of linoleic acid and other polyunsaturated fatty acids are influenced both by maternal diet and by maternal body fat composition, all human milk is rich in long-chained polyunsaturated fatty acids, which are important in brain development and myelinization. Most breast-milk substitutes contain little or none of these (62–64), although in 1989 some manufacturers planned to add them. Cow's milk has higher concentrations of short- and medium-chained fatty acids which, in the 1960s and 1970s, sometimes combined with the higher casein content of earlier breast-milk substitutes to form insoluble soaps responsible for milk bolus obstruction and intestinal perforation in term infants. Regrettably, this problem has recently re-emerged in sick preterm infants being fed high-density breast-milk substitutes (65, 66).

Among the polyunsaturated fatty acids, arachidonic and linoleic acids are particularly important. Arachidonic acid is considered essential during infancy because linoleic acid in vivo is not as readily convertible into arachidonic acid. The content of these two fatty acids is about four times higher in human than in cow's milk (0.4 g and 0.1 g/100 ml, respectively). Prostaglandins, whose synthesis is dependent on the availability of these essential fatty acids, are widely distributed in the gastrointestinal tract (67). They affect a variety of physiological functions that enhance digestion as well as the maturation of intestinal cells, and thus contribute to the overall host defence mechanisms. Human milk can contain significant quantities of prostaglandins (68); breast-milk substitutes contain none. Human milk also contains other lipid-associated antiviral compounds.

While glucose is the fetus' main energy source, the infant is highly dependent on fats for energy; breast milk provides 35–50% of daily intake in the form of fats. The infant begins to consume this high-fat diet at a time when both pancreatic lipase secretion and the efficiency of bile salt conjugation are immature (69). Their immaturity is partially compensated for by lingual and gastric lipases, but the presence of a non-specific lipase in human milk is particularly significant. This enzyme is activated by bile salts in the duodenum and thus contributes to the infant's fat digestion, which is a feature that is absent from most other milks. In fact, humans and gorillas are the only two mammals that provide their offspring with both a substrate and its enzyme in the same fluid. When fresh breast milk is the main source of fat, it is estimated that the bile salt-stimulated lipase will contribute to the digestion of 30–40% of triglycerides within 2 hours. This process proceeds in vitro as well as in vivo. It is particularly important in the feeding of preterm infants, whose bile salt and pancreatic lipase production is even more depressed (see chapter 5). However, unheated breast milk should be used since milk lipase is destroyed by heating (70). Lipase is only one of dozens of enzymes present in human milk (see below), and it acts as a metabolic modulator for the infant in ways that no other food can mimic.

Human milk is uniformly rich in cholesterol, the importance of which is still not understood. There is conflicting evidence from laboratory animals which suggests that early exposure to cholesterol may affect adult handling of this important lipid. It is not known whether the presence or absence of bovine cholesterol in breast-milk substitutes is an advantage to the artificially fed infant. Without further research in this area, reliable dietary guidelines for children under two years of age cannot be formulated, despite accumulating evidence suggesting that dietary factors in infancy are involved in the later development of cardiovascular disease (71) (see chapter 4).

Lactose

Lactose is human milk's major carbohydrate, although small amounts of galactose, fructose, and other oligosaccharides are also present. It is a sugar found only in milk, and human milk contains the highest concentrations (an average of 4% in colostrum, increasing to 7% in mature milk). Lactose appears to be a specific nutrient for infancy, since the enzyme lactase is found only in infant mammals. Lactase persists among Europeans and some other populations, but most people do not tolerate lactose after middle childhood; foods containing lactose can thus cause intestinal disturbance.

Lactose furnishes about 40% of energy needs but also has other functions. It is metabolized into glucose (used for energy) and galactose, a constituent of the galactolipids needed for the development of the central nervous system. It facilitates calcium and iron absorption, and promotes intestinal colonization with *Lactobacillus bifidus*. These fermentative bacteria promote an acidic milieu in the gastrointestinal tract, inhibiting the growth of pathogenic bacteria, fungi and parasites. The growth of *L. bifidus* is further encouraged by the presence in human milk of a nitrogen-containing carbohydrate, the bifidus factor, which is not found in bovine-milk derivatives. Food supplements given in the first days after birth interfere with this protective mechanism (*72*). Ruminant animals require a different gut flora and ecology; artificially fed infants are thus colonized predominantly with coliform and putrefactive bacteria, and their stools have a higher pH value. It is usual to find reducing substances such as sugars in the stools of healthy breast-fed infants; they contribute to maintaining the acid environment that retards the growth of pathogens. In contrast, the delayed gut transit time of industrially prepared milks (*73*) permits almost total metabolism of these sugars.

Primary lactose intolerance is a rare congenital anomaly (see below). Varying degrees of temporary lactose intolerance can occur with any condition that damages the intestinal brush border and results in a loss of lactase (e.g., rotavirus, *Giardia lamblia*, or cow's-milk protein intolerance). Without the enzyme to metabolize it, lactose is fermented by gut bacteria, producing an extremely acid stool, which can itself further damage the brush border. The infant experiences abdominal pain; passes frequent, frothy, liquid stools; and, in extreme cases, may fail to thrive or be at risk of dehydration. Only rarely is it necessary to briefly interrupt breast-feeding; indeed, breast-feeding should almost always continue, and even increase, during periods of diarrhoea (see chapter 6).

Another situation of relative lactose intolerance has recently been postulated, the cure for which is a simple change in breast-feeding management. Mothers may find that they have irritable, unsettled, "colicky" babies whose stools are frequent and liquid, who pass urine and regurgitate frequently, but who are otherwise thriving; they may be gaining weight well or poorly. It is hypothesized that when a mother, who typically has more than enough milk, fails to allow her infant enough time at the first breast and, instead, changes sides after a pre-determined period, the infant may ingest a feed that is too high in lactose and too low in fat (*74*). Lactose intolerance is sometimes resolved within 24 hours if a mother lets her infant "finish" the first breast before offering the second when it is clear that the infant is not satisfied. After a day or two of feeding by choice from one breast, supply will diminish and the infant will insist

on feeding from both breasts at each feed, but without the symptoms of apparent lactose intolerance. This theory is supported by the observation that many such unsettled infants have higher than average breath-hydrogen levels (*75*).

Despite the apparent importance of lactose for normal infants, not all breast-milk substitutes contain this carbohydrate. This is understandable in the case of formulas designed for short-term therapeutic use by lactose-intolerant infants. The short- and long-term consequences of feeding lactose-free substitutes to healthy infants from birth are unknown. Likewise, the role of the other oligosaccharides in human milk is under-researched, although they make up 25% of colostrum, and at least one—the carbohydrate known as the bifidus factor—prevents microbial colonization.

Vitamins

Vitamin concentrations in human milk are almost always adequate for infant needs, although they can vary with maternal intake. Given the variability of fat concentrations in human milk, and the relationship of fat to maternal diet, infant intakes of fat-soluble vitamins can differ markedly. The concentration of vitamin A in human milk is higher than in cow's milk except among deficient populations (*76*), and there is twice the amount in colostrum than in mature milk. In the second year of life, vitmin A deficiency is more common among infants weaned early than among those who are still breast-fed.

In the immediate post-partum period the concentration of vitamin K is higher in colostrum and early breast milk (*77*) than in later milk. However, after two weeks vitamin K-supplying intestinal flora will be established in breast-fed infants. Where infants are deprived of colostrum, or of hindmilk, the risk of haemorrhagic disease is greater than in artificially fed infants, unless vitamin K is provided soon after birth. Oral doses are used by some clinicians (see chapter 3); research into their efficacy would benefit those infants in situations where injections are not desirable.

The vitamin E content of human milk usually meets the needs of the infant unless a mother is consuming excess amounts of polyunsaturated fats without a concomitant increase in vitamin E intake.

The vitamin D content of human milk is low (an average of 0.15 µg/100 ml), and for some years it was considered insufficient to meet the needs of the infant, even though exclusively breast-fed infants do not routinely develop a deficiency. Later, the presence of water-soluble vitamin D in the aqueous phase of milk was discovered in concentrations as high as 0.88 µg/

100 ml (78). Debate ensued as to the biological significance of this water-soluble vitamin D, and it is now understood that the optimal route for vitamin D ingestion in humans is not the gastrointestinal tract, which may permit toxic amounts to be absorbed. Rather, the skin is the human organ designed, in the presence of sunlight, both to manufacture vitamin D in potentially vast quantities and to prevent the absorption of more than the body can safely use and store. It takes only brief exposure to sunlight to produce sufficient vitamin D; to satisfy a week's requirements for white infants in a midwestern US city the exposure time is 10 minutes unclothed or 30 minutes with only the head and hands exposed (79). The only groups at risk of vitamin D deficiency are women and children who do not eat marine oils and who are totally covered and not exposed to daylight.

Variations in water-soluble vitamins can occur, depending on the maternal diet, but levels are generally more than ample in the milk of well-nourished mothers. Case-reports of deficiencies in infants are rare, even among poorly nourished women or vegan women who are more at risk of vitamin B deficiencies. The concentration of vitamin B_{12} is very low in human milk, but its bioavailability is enhanced by a specific transfer factor. Concentration of niacin, folic acid, and ascorbic acid is generally higher than in the milk of ruminants. Special care is required in environments where a deficiency in some vitamins is endemic, for example vitamin A or thiamine (80). Long-term users of oral contraceptives may also have lower levels of vitamin B_6 in their milk. Although mothers may fail to demonstrate clinical signs, their milk can still be deficient in these vitamins with adverse consequences for their infants. Improving the mother's diet, which is a priority in its own right, is the most cost-effective way of preventing any vitamin deficiency in the breast-fed infant.

Minerals

The concentration of most minerals in breast milk, e.g., calcium, iron, phosphorus, magnesium, zinc, potassium, and fluoride, will not be significantly affected by maternal diet. Compensatory mechanisms, such as decreased urinary calcium excretion, come into play, and only in extreme cases will a mother's own reserves or tissues be significantly depleted. In these cases the post-lactational recovery period is of great importance. In the case of fluoride, it appears that the breast inhibits passage into the milk of any but trace amounts (81).

Mineral concentrations are lower in human milk than in any breast-milk substitute, and are thus better adapted to the infant's nutritional requirements and metabolic capacities. Calcium is more efficiently absorbed because of human milk's high calcium:phosphorus ratio (2:1). The higher phosphorus concentration of cow's milk leads to preferential absorption of phosphorus and is responsible for neonatal hypocalcaemia, which is more common among artificially than breast-fed infants. Calcium availability from cow's milk is decreased even further by the formation of insoluble calcium soaps in the gut, which can cause intestinal obstruction and perforation (see above). The calcium:phosphorus ratio of breast-milk substitutes has generally been modified to improve calcium absorption, although their range is still considerable.

Similarly, the high bioavailability of human-milk iron is the result of a series of complex interactions between the components of breast milk and the infant's body. The higher acidity of the gastrointestinal tract; the presence of appropriate levels of zinc and copper; the transfer factor lactoferrin, which prevents iron from being available to intestinal bacteria and releases it only when specific receptors unlock the lactoferrin molecule—all these factors are important to increase iron absorption. Up to 70% of breast-milk iron is absorbed, compared with 30% in cow's milk and only 10% in breast-milk substitutes (82). To compensate, large amounts of supplemental iron have to be added to substitutes, which favours the development of pathogenic gut bacteria.

Iron-deficiency anaemia is extremely rare in infants fed only breast milk during the first 6–8 months of life. Indeed, healthy infants born at term to well-nourished mothers have sufficient hepatic iron stores to meet their needs for the better part of the first year (83). Early introduction of other foods in the diet of the breast-fed infant can alter this picture, however (see chapter 4). It has been shown, for example, that pears chelate breast-milk iron, making it insoluble and rendering it unavailable to the infant (84). Even supplemental iron may cause problems by saturating lactoferrin, thus decreasing its bacteriostatic effect, and encouraging the growth of pathogens, some of which can cause sufficient gut damage and microscopic bleeding to produce iron-deficiency anaemia (85). At the same time, providing additional iron can reduce zinc or copper absorption. While there are specific indications for infant iron supplementation, e.g., extreme prematurity and considerable neonatal blood loss, they are not without risk. See chapter 5.

In populations where the prevalence of iron deficiency is high there are many women who enter pregnancy already suffering from various degrees of anaemia. In such situations full therapeutic doses of a well absorbed iron salt are obviously needed (86). On the other hand, in many developed countries most women enter pregnancy not only with normal haemoglobin concentrations but also with a reserve of iron of 200–300 mg. The supplementation required in such instances is less, since all that is required is a daily dose of iron sufficient to meet the increased needs of pregnancy, which in the second and third trimesters is about 5–6 mg daily (86). More study is needed on the effect of routine iron supplementation during pregnancy of healthy, non-anaemic women; one recent study shows that both folate and iron-folate supplements decreased the maternal serum zinc levels within 24 hours (87).

The above recommendations, however, relate exclusively to the iron status of the mother. Most studies, based either on the measurement of ferritin in the newborn (88, 89) or the later development of anaemia (90, 91) suggest that iron status at birth is little dependent on the iron nutrition of the mother. Similarly, there is no evidence that maternal iron status bears any relationship to the iron-content of breast milk (83).

Zinc is essential to enzyme structure and function, growth, and cellular immunity. The amounts of zinc in human milk are small but sufficient to meet the needs of infants without disturbing copper and iron absorption; its bioavailability is high compared with the zinc added to breast-milk substitutes. Human milk is therapeutic in cases of acrodermatitis enteropathica, which is a disease associated with zinc deficiency. Although occasionally reported in breast-fed infants, this condition is far more common among the artificially fed. The level of available zinc varies widely in breast-milk substitutes, and soya formulas have been found to be deficient in this regard (92). High zinc:copper ratios have been associated with coronary heart disease; the corresponding ratio in breast milk is lower than that of the usual substitutes.

Trace elements

Once again there are substantial differences between trace elements in human milk and any substitute; only a few can be mentioned in a review of this nature. In general, the breast-fed infant is at little risk of either a deficiency or an excess of trace elements. Copper, cobalt and selenium levels in human milk are generally higher than in cow's milk. Enhanced bioavailability of breast-milk copper results from its binding with proteins of low relative molecular mass. Copper deficiency, resulting in a hypochromic microcytic anaemia and neurological disturbances, occurs only in artificially fed infants (93, 94). At three months of age, selenium status is better in exclusively breast-fed than in mixed or artificially fed infants (95). Breast-milk selenium levels are slightly lower in areas where soils are selenium-deficient. However, bovine

milk selenium is affected even more markedly by dietary intake, varying by as much as 100-fold. There is considerable discussion about the appropriate level of selenium in breast-milk substitutes (96). Levels of chromium (97), manganese (98) and aluminium (99) may be up to 100 times greater than in human milk, and some effects on later learning and on bone growth have been postulated. Recently, lead and cadmium have been shown to contaminate formulas still stored in soldered cans (100). Dietary lead intake is much lower in breast-fed infants, even where drinking-water exceeds the WHO standard (0.1 μg lead per ml) (101). Iodine can be concentrated in milk. In addition, the topical use of iodine (e.g., in skin washes) can affect the breast-fed infant's thyroid function (102).

With minerals as with other nutrients, there are many significant differences between human milk and substitutes. Great advances in knowledge about mineral interactions and bioavailability have occurred in the last decade (103). It is now recognized that the ability of breast-milk substitutes to provide adequate levels of nutrients cannot be predicted from their compositional analysis alone, and that growth by itself is not a sufficiently sensitive indicator of all possible adverse outcomes due to deficiency or excess. Further study is required on these and other components, including nickel, vanadium, tin, silicon, arsenic and cadmium.

Other substances

Human milk is not only a source of nutrients uniquely adapted to the infant's metabolic capacities; recent research has indicated that it may even exercise a degree of control over metabolism, from the subtleties of cell division to infant behaviour (104), as well as over the development and maintenance of breast function. Some hormones (105) present in milk have already been mentioned (oxytocin, prolactin, adrenal and ovarian steroids, and prostaglandins). A full list would also include Gn-RH (gonadotropin-releasing hormone), GRF (growth hormone releasing factor), insulin, somatostatin, relaxin, calcitonin, and neurotensin at levels greater than those in maternal blood; and TRH (thyrotropin-releasing hormone), TSH (thyroid-stimulating hormone), thyroxine, triiodothyronine, erythropoietin, and bombesin at levels less than in maternal sera. The evidence that endocrine responses differ between breast-fed and artificially fed infants is reviewed elsewhere (106). In addition, hormonal release may be influenced by compounds in milk such as the human beta-casomorphins, which are peptides with opioid activity that may also affect the neonatal central nervous system. Nucleotides (affecting fat absorption) and numerous growth factors are present in human milk. The latter include epidermal growth factor (EGF), insulin-like growth factor (IGF-I), human milk growth factors (HMGF-I, II, and III), and nerve growth factor (NGF). Their role in the development of the infant is only just beginning to be elucidated (107).

The dozens of enzymes in human milk have a multi-functional origin. Some reflect the physiological changes occurring in the breasts; others are important for neonatal development (protcolytic enzymes, peroxidase, lysozyme, xanthine oxidase); still others augment the infant's own digestive enzymes (alpha-amylase and bile salt-stimulated lipase). Many are found in much higher concentrations in colostrum than in mature milk, e.g., lysozyme whose concentration is about 5000 times greater in human than in cow's milk. This enzyme is bacteriolytic against Gram-positive bacteria and may also afford specific protection against some viruses. Other enzymes are believed to have direct immunological functions, while some may be acting indirectly by promoting cell maturation (108, 109).

Immunological qualities of breast milk

Human milk is much more than a simple collection of nutrients; it is a living substance of great biological complexity that is both actively protective and immunomodulatory. It not only provides unique protection against infections and allergies (110–112), but it also stimulates the appropriate development of the infant's own immune system. In addition, it contains many anti-inflammatory components whose functions are not fully understood (113). The most immediately apparent result is decreased infant morbidity and mortality, compared with infants who are artificially fed, the impact of which is particularly dramatic in poor communities (114, 115). However, the immunological benefits of breast milk are no less real among relatively affluent populations, (116, 117). For example, recent research indicates that there are subtle immunological risks among artificially fed, compared with breast-fed, infants in wealthier communities where there is apparently a greater incidence in childhood of otitis media (118), coeliac disease (119), Crohn disease (120), diabetes (121), and cancer (122), in addition to problems due to the mechanics of artificial feeding, such as orthodontic defect (123). Decreased morbidity among breast-fed infants in industrialized countries has remained constant even during periods when it was the less privileged who breast-fed (124).

The methodological flaws of past studies of the protective effect of breast milk in developed countries have served to confuse the issue. Given the impor-

tance of gut flora in disease, it is critical to distinguish carefully *inter alia* between infants who have received only breast milk from birth, infants receiving supplementary foods neonatally and only breast milk thereafter, infants who are breast-fed but supplemented from birth with breast-milk substitutes, and infants who are artificially fed from birth (125). In studies designed to assess the health effects of infant feeding, all other fluids and solids given to the infant need to be recorded.

A recent study in Dundee, Scotland, followed 674 mother–infant pairs for two years in an effort to overcome these methodological flaws. It was found that the infants who were breast fed for 3 months or more had substantially less gastrointestinal illness during the first year of life than the infants who were bottle-fed from birth or completely weaned at an early stage. This reduction in illness, which was found whether or not supplements were introduced before 13 weeks, was maintained beyond the point of breast-feeding itself and was accompanied by a reduction in the rate of hospital admission. By contrast, infants who were breast-fed for less than 13 weeks had rates of gastrointestinal illness similar to those observed in bottle-fed infants (126).

The protection afforded by breast-feeding is most evident in early life and continues in proportion to the frequency and duration of breast-feeding. The neonate must contend with a number of immediate problems at birth, including colonization of the intestines with microorganisms, the toxins produced by the microorganisms, and the ingestion of macromolecular antigens; all three can cause pathological reactions if permitted to penetrate the intestinal barrier. The intestinal host defence mechanisms are immature at birth; thereafter, the wealth of immune substances and growth factors in colostrum and breast milk protect the intestinal mucosa against penetration, modify the intestinal luminal environment to suppress the growth of some pathogenic microorganisms while killing others, stimulate epithelial maturation, and enhance digestive enzyme production (127).

The anti-infective properties in colostrum and breast milk have both soluble and cellular components (128). The soluble components include immunoglobulins (IgA, IgM, IgG) as well as lysozymes and other enzymes, lactoferrin, the bifidus factor, and other immunoregulatory substances (39, 48). The cellular components include macrophages (which contain IgA, lysozymes and lactoferrin), lymphocytes, neutrophil granulocytes, and epithelial cells. While the concentration of these constituents is very high in colostrum, it decreases in mature milk. However, because decreased concentration is compensated for by increasing milk volume, infant intakes remain more or less constant throughout lactation (see Table 2.1).

Table 2.1: **Distribution of immunoglobulins and other soluble substances in the colostrum and milk delivered to the breast-fed infant during a 24-hour period**[a]

Soluble product	Concentration in mg/day at postpartum:			
	< 1 week	1–2 weeks	3–4 weeks	> 4 weeks
IgG	50	25	25	10
IgA	5000	1000	1000	1000
IgM	70	30	15	10
Lysozyme	50	60	60	100
Lactoferrin	1500	2000	2000	1200

[a] Reference 129.

The protection afforded the infant is substantial. Calculated on a per/kg body-weight basis, it has been estimated that a fully breast-fed infant receives 0.5 g secretory IgA (SIgA) per day, which is about 50 times the globulin dose given to a patient with hypo-globulinaemia. SIgA is the most important globulin fraction; it is produced by the subepithelial plasma cells of the intestinal tract except during the first 4–6 weeks of life (or even longer in allergic individuals) when infants need to obtain it from breast milk. SIgA is also produced in the mammary gland (130). It is resistant to proteolytic enzymes and low pH, and considerable amounts of ingested SIgA can be recovered in an infant's stool (131). Soluble IgA covers the infant's intestinal mucosa like "white paint", rendering it impermeable to pathogens. It is believed that the SIgA antibodies bind toxins, bacteria and macromolecular antigens, thus preventing their access to the epithelium. Breast milk also stimulates the infant's own production of SIgA (132, 133).

Other breast-milk components also have an immunological role. Lactoferrin is an unsaturated, iron-binding glycoprotein that competes for iron with iron-dependent microorganisms, and is thus bacteriostatic. Like SIgA, lactoferrin is resistant to proteolytic activity. As mentioned earlier, the bifidus factor occurring in fresh colostrum and breast milk is a nitrogen-containing carbohydrate that is easily destroyed by heat (69); it promotes intestinal colonization with lactobacilli in the presence of lactose. The resulting low pH in the intestinal lumen inhibits the growth of both E. coli, Gram-negative bacteria, and fungi such as Candida albicans. A similarly low pH in the stomach may be of particular importance to the premature and low-birth-weight infant (134, 135) (see chapter 5). The growth of pathogens in the

stomach may lead to the emptying into the intestines of highly contaminated feeds (136), and increased risk of potentially fatal disorders such as necrotizing enterocolitis, which occurs only rarely in infants fed only human milk from birth. For example, in a neonatal unit in Helsinki, a study of over 7000 sick infants found only 5 cases, of whom 3 were full-term infants after exchange transfusions. All infants that died were autopsied; all premature infants were radiologically screened (136). A neonatal unit in Manila (R. Gonzales, personal communication, 1989) has not had a single case since converting to human-milk feeding; maternity hospitals in Stockholm (136) and Oslo (R. Lindemann, personal communication, 1989) report similar findings.

Recent research indicates the presence in human milk of other factors having specific immunological functions. Indeed, it is now clear that there is a broncho-mammary and an entero-mammary circulation, which ensures that every pathogen that challenges a mother stimulates the production of specific antibodies that are present in the milk her infant receives. Breast milk has been shown to be active, in vitro, against many pathogens (137) (see Tables 2.2 to 2.4) and specific protection against many of these (including rotavirus (138) and G. lamblia (139, 140)) is provided to the infant. Breast milk also contains viral fragments that cannot be replicated, but which stimulate antibody responses in infants, effectively immunizing them before exposure to the active agent, or enhancing their response. Now that PCR (polymerase chain-reaction) tests are available, which can amplify and detect traces of certain viruses, it should be borne in mind that proof of the presence of antigenic fragments reveals little about their function in milk. There has been no study to date of the potential preventive or therapeutic roles of human milk in HIV infection (see chapter 3).

The activity of the cellular components of breast milk is not yet well understood. Macrophages are in highest concentration, followed by lymphocytes and neutrophil granulocytes. These cells help to prevent infection both by phagocytosis and by secretion of immune substances having some degree of specificity for those microorganisms with which the mother is in contact (130).

Effects on mothers

Breast-milk quantity

The volume of breast milk varies according to infant demand, the frequency of breast-feeding, the stage of lactation, and glandular capacity. It is only in cases of extreme deprivation that a mother's nutritional status may have an adverse effect on milk volume. In

Table 2.2: **Antibacterial factors found in human milk**[a]

Factor	Shown, *in vitro*, to be active against:	Effect of heat
Secretory IgA	*E. coli* (also pili and capsular antigens), *C. tetani*, *C. diphtheriae*, *K. pneumoniae*, *Salmonella* (6 groups), *Shigella* (2 groups), *Streptococcus*, *S. mutans*, *S. sanguis*, *S. mitis*, *S. salivarius*, *S. pneumoniae*, *C. burnetti*, *H. influenzae* *E. coli* enterotoxin, *V. cholerae* enterotoxin, *C. difficile* toxins, *H. influenzae* capsule	Stable at 56°C for 30 min; some loss (0–30%) at 62.5°C for 30 min; destroyed by boiling
IgM, IgG	*V. cholerae* lipopolysaccharide; *F. coli*	IgM destroyed and IgG decreased by a third at 62.5°C for 30 min
IgD	*E. coli*	
Bifidobacterium bifidum growth z factor	Enterobacteriacea, enteric pathogens	Stable to boiling
Factor binding proteins (zinc, vitamin B_{12}, folate)	Dependent *E. coli*	Destroyed by boiling
Complement C1–C9 (mainly C3 and C4)	Effect not known	Destroyed by heating at 56°C for 30 min
Lactoferrin	*E. coli*	Two-thirds destroyed at 62.5°C for 30 min
Lactoperoxidase	*Streptococcus*, *Pseudomonas*, *E. coli*, *S. typhimurium*	Destroyed by boiling
Lysozyme	*E. coli*, *Salmonella*, *Micrococcus lysodeikticus*	Some loss (0–23%) at 62.5°C for 30 min; essentially destroyed by boiling for 15 min
Unidentified factors	*S. aureus*; *C. difficile* toxin B	Stable at autoclaving; stable at 56°C for 30 min
Carbohydrate	*E. coli* enterotoxin	Stable at 85°C for 30 min
Lipid	*S. aureus*	Stable to boiling
Ganglioside (GMI like)	*E. coli* enterotoxin, *V. cholerae* enterotoxin	Stable to boiling
Glycoproteins (receptor-like) + oligosaccharides	*V. cholerae*	Stable to boiling for 15 min
Analogues of epithelial cell receptors (oligosaccharides)	*S. pneumoniae*, *H. influenzae*	Stable to boiling
Milk cells (macrophages, neutrophils, B and T lymphocytes)	By phagocytosis and killing: *E. coli*. *S. aureus*, *S. enteritidis*. By sensitized lymphocytes: *E. coli* By phagocytosis: *C. albicans*, *E. coli*. Lymphocyte stimulation: *E. coli* K antigen, tuberculin PPD. Monocyte chemotactic factor production: PPD	Destroyed at 62.5°C for 30 min

[a] Reference *137*.

the WHO study concerning the quantity and quality of breast milk (*40*), a "threshold effect", after which breast-milk volume decreased, was observed among rural mothers in Zaire who had less than 30 g/l serum albumin levels (normal levels are 35–45 g/l). Except for this finding, no correlation was established between milk volume and maternal anthropometric characteristics, serum protein and albumin levels, and erythrocyte and haemoglobin counts. However, mothers in Sweden had a significantly higher milk volume during the first four months of lactation. The milk volume per 15 minutes of sucking was also higher among Hungarian and Swedish mothers, two groups enjoying high socioeconomic standards compared to mothers in Guatemala, the Philippines and Zaire.

Milk volume does not correlate with energy content, however; some mothers who are over-producing milk find that once the intake volume is reduced, their infants feed for longer periods at less-frequent intervals and put on more weight. In addition, recent research has demonstrated that, when milk volume drops, the milk tends to become more energy-dense, at the expense of maternal body stores if need be. Data about breast-milk volume demonstrate little about the energy value of the milk provided, however. Infants thrive on widely different volumes and energy intakes.

Table 2.3: **Antiviral factors found in human milk**[a]

Factor	Shown, *in vitro*, to be active against:	Effect of heat
Secretory IgA	Poliovirus types 1, 2, 3. Coxsackie types A9, B3, B5, echovirus types 6, 9. Semliki Forest virus, Ross River virus, rotavirus, cytomegalovirus, reovirus type 3, rubella virus, herpes simplex virus, mumps virus, influenza virus, respiratory syncytial virus	Stable at 56°C for 30 min; some loss (0–30%) at 62.5°C for 30 min; destroyed by boiling
IgM, IgG	Rubella virus, cytomegalovirus, respiratory syncytial virus	IgM destroyed and IgG decreased by a third at 62.5°C for 30 min
Lipid (unsaturated fatty acids and monoglycerides)	Herpes simplex virus, Semliki Forest virus, influenza virus, dengue, Ross River virus, Japanese B encephalitis virus, Sindbis virus, West Nile virus	Stable to boiling for 30 min
Non-immunoglobulin macromolecules	Herpes simplex virus, vesicular stomatitis virus, Coxsackie B4 virus, Semliki Forest virus, reovirus 3, poliotype 2, cytomegalovirus, respiratory syncytial virus, rotavirus	Most stable at 56°C for 30 min and destroyed by boiling
α_2-macroglobulin (like)	Influenza virus haemagglutinin, parainfluenza virus haemagglutin	Stable to boiling for 15 min
Ribonuclease	Murine leukaemia virus	Stable at 62.5°C for 30 min
Haemagglutinin inhibitors	Influenza and mumps viruses	Destroyed by boiling
Milk cells	Induced interferon: virus or PHA Induced lymphokine (LDCF): phytohaemagglutinin (PHA) Induced cytokine: by herpes simplex virus Lymphocyte stimulation: cytomegalovirus, rubella, herpes, measles, mumps, respiratory syncytial viruses	Destroyed at 62.5°C for 30 min

[a] Reference *137*

Of considerable significance are recent findings that thriving infants, who are fed only breast milk by well-nourished mothers, regulate their own intake within a wide range; that this intake volume is well within the lactational capacity of even poorly nourished women; and that the intake volume is relatively stable between one and four months of age (*141*). In contrast, infants fed only breast-milk substitutes increase their intake volume during the same period by an average of an additional 200 ml/day (*142*). The metabolic consequences of this greater intake as well as its possible later significance for such diet-related problems as obesity are unknown (see chapter 4).

Nutritional requirements of lactating mothers

Women's nutritional requirements during lactation vary widely. Energy is needed to cover the energy content of the milk secreted, plus the energy required to produce it. The nutritional cost to the mother in proteins, vitamins and minerals is considerable (*143*), and unless these additional energy and nutrient requirements are met, lactation will take place at the expense of maternal tissues. As previously discussed, changes in metabolic efficiency during pregnancy provide for the anticipated expenditures of lactation. An adequately nourished mother accumulates nutrient stores during pregnancy that are used to compensate for her higher requirements during the first months of lactation.

The extent of those requirements has been the subject of considerable discussion (see chapter 1). Since 1981, much work has gone into the many methodological problems of determining what constitutes a representative breast-milk sample (*144*). First, the estimated average caloric value of breast milk has been progressively revised downwards (from

Table 2.4: **Antiparasite factors found in human milk**[a]

Factor	Shown, *in vitro*, to be active against:	Effect of heat
Secretory IgA	G. lamblia E. histolytica S. mansoni Cryptosporidium	Stable at 56°C for 30 min, some loss (0–30%) at 62.5°C for 30 min, destroyed by boiling
Lipid (free)	G. lamblia E. histolytica T. vaginalis	Stable to boiling
Unidentified	T. rhodesiense	

[a] Reference *137*.

70 to 65 kcal), which affects the calculation of what energy is required both to replace and to produce breast milk. Second, it appears that the metabolic efficiency of women is considerably improved during lactation, so that maternal food intake is more effectively utilized than normally (145).

Studies of women whose milk is their infants' sole source of nourishment, and who have access to as much extra food as they wish, have shown very different patterns of caloric intake during lactation. Almost none met the 1981 guidelines (146), including those women whose weight remained stable and whose infants were obviously thriving. Some women do not lose weight despite intakes that are theoretically inadequate to sustain full lactation. Similarly, substantial supplementation (roughly 750 kcal added to a normal daily intake of only 1500 kcal) given to undernourished Gambian women made no difference in their milk output (2); mean milk intakes of infants were 750 ml from both Gambian and English mothers of 3-month-old infants, which closely matches data regarding infants in Texas (USA) who were fed only breast milk (142). While there may be selective depletion of adequately nourished mothers' nutrient stores during lactation, there is little evidence that this is clinically significant in a range of normal circumstances. Research into the late-lactation and post-lactation recovery of these body stores suggests enhanced uptake at these times and during a subsequent pregnancy; however, more work is required to throw light on the ideal inter-birth interval for maternal recovery of lactational losses.

There do seem to be a number of compensatory mechanisms that allow for lactation to continue with much lower energy and nutrient intakes, or even with no caloric increase over the diet of the non-pregnant, non-lactating woman. This does not mean, of course, that lactating women in general do not need to increase their food intakes; rather, it suggests that nutritional status before and during pregnancy plays an important role in lactation performance. However, because of the very wide differences between individuals in nutritional status, metabolic efficiency, and energy expenditure, no universal statement as to maternal nutritional needs can be made. Estimates of "average need" have been revised downwards in recent years (see chapter 1). The amount of physical exertion in a mother's daily routine obviously affects any such calculation.

A mixed and varied diet, which satisfies normal requirements during the non-pregnant and non-lactating period, will usually cover the extra needs for lactation if total intake is increased to satisfy additional energy needs. Monitoring maternal weight provides some guide as to the adequacy of a mother's energy intake. Women around the world breast-feed successfully on many different, and frequently less-than-optimal, diets. Little work has been done to define what would constitute an optimal lactation diet; the key area of interest at present would appear to be the optimal pattern of fatty acid intake.

Greatly increased fluid intake has been frequently stressed in breast-feeding literature. However there is no evidence that either restricting or increasing fluid intake affects lactation success (147). Where maternal fluid intake is deficient, the urine will become concentrated and a mother will be thirsty. Women should drink amounts sufficient to satisfy thirst and to keep their urine dilute.

Lactation and contraception

The full importance of lactation as the world's most significant contraceptive (148) can only be mentioned briefly in this review of lactation. A consensus statement (149) adopted recently summarized what is now known about the conditions under which breast-feeding can be used as a safe and effective contraceptive. The maximum birth-spacing effect is achieved when an infant is fully or nearly fully breast-fed and a mother consequently remains amenorrhoeic. When these two conditions are fulfilled breast-feeding provides more than 98% protection in the first six months postpartum. After six months, or when breast milk is supplemented, or menses return, the risk of pregnancy increases, although it remains low while breast-feeding continues at much the same level. See also chapter 3.

In any discussion of infant feeding, it is important to understand the impact of breast-feeding on the time interval between births and the consequences where providing optimal nutrition for the mother, her infant and any subsequent children are concerned. It is significant that the period of full breast-feeding required to maximize the mother's protection against a subsequent pregnancy, without need for artificial means of contraception is identical to the period of full breast-feeding required to maximize the infant's protection against allergic and infectious disease. Prolonged amenorrhoea also permits the mother to recover her iron stores, which enhances her immune and nutritional status as well as the prospects for providing adequate nutrition for any future fetus.

Résumé

La lactation

La lactation est le moyen le plus efficace du point de vue énergétique pour satisfaire les besoins diététiques des jeunes mammifères, le lait de leur mère leur assurant en outre une protection active. Beaucoup de questions sur la physiologie de la lactation chez la femme demandent des réponses. On présente ici un résumé du développement de la glande mammaire depuis le stade embryologique jusqu'à sa complète maturité et l'on insiste sur les changements qui se produisent au niveau du mamelon et du sein lui-même pendant la grossesse et à terme. Il existe en effet une relation entre l'épaisseur des tissus qui entourent le mamelon, la rétractilité de celui-ci et la capacité de l'enfant à bien téter.

Les phénomènes hormonaux qui se produisent pendant la grossesse sont ensuite décrits. Le rôle de la prolactine dans le développement du sein est discuté ainsi que celui des œstrogènes sur le développement des alvéoles. Les différentes phases de la lactogenèse sont décrites ainsi que la séquence selon laquelle prolactine et ocytocine interviennent. Dès la naissance de grandes quantités de lait sont produites et les tétées vont stimuler la sécrétion de prolactine favorisant la lactogenèse. Pour le maintien de la lactation, il est essentiel que la manière d'alimenter le nourrisson respecte certaines conditions. Il faut que le sein soit pris efficacement, fréquemment et pendant des périodes suffisamment longues pour que soit prévenue, entre autres, la constitution de complexes métaboliques peptidiques inhibiteurs de la lactation.

Après la description des réflexes maternels de production et d'éjection du lait, ce sont les réflexes complémentaires existant chez le nourrisson qui sont analysés. Chez le nouveau-né normal tous ces réflexes sont présents dès la naissance et demandent à être consolidés par des comportements acquis dans la période qui suit. Pour initier avec succès l'allaitement maternel il faudrait que les nouveaux-nés puissent prendre le sein dans l'heure qui suit la naissance, au moment où à la fois leurs réflexes et la sensibilité de la mère à tous les stimuli sont les plus forts. Pour maintenir avec succès cet allaitement il faut que tous les facteurs qui pourraient diminuer la qualité de la succion de l'enfant soient, dans la mesure du possible, éliminés.

La composition du lait maternel est décrite en détail depuis le stade du colostrum jusqu'à sa maturation complète. Il s'agit d'un processus qui peut présenter des variations dépendant non seulement de facteurs strictement maternels mais aussi de la relation mère-enfant. D'un point de vue immunologique le lait de la mère non seulement apporte une protection contre infections et allergies mais aussi stimule le développement du système immunitaire de l'enfant.

La morbidité générale a toujours été plus basse chez les enfants nourris au sein dans les pays industrialisés même au cours de périodes où ce mode d'allaitement prédominait parmi les groupes les plus défavorisés. Une étude récente réalisée à Dundee, Ecosse a fait la preuve de la supériorité du lait maternel dans la protection contre les affections gastro-entéritiques dans la population objet de l'enquête. Cette étude a éliminé la plupart des causes d'erreurs qui avaient biaisé les études antérieures les rendant peu concluantes.

La quantité de lait produite varie en fonction de la demande de l'enfant, de la fréquence des tétées, du stade de la lactation et de la capacité de la glande. Ce n'est que dans les cas de privations extrêmes que l'état nutritionnel de la mère peut retentir négativement sur le volume du lait. Des mécanismes compensatoires interviennent qui permettent à la lactation de se maintenir avec des apports énergétiques relativement bas; ce qui explique qu'il est difficile de fixer de manière précise les besoins nutritionnels des femmes allaitantes (voir chapitre 1). Leur état nutritionnel avant et durant la grossesse joue par ailleurs un rôle important.

Enfin l'allaitement maternel en tant que moyen de contraception naturel est mentionné. L'aménorrhée lactationnelle permet un espacement des naissances et l'allaitement maternel assure une protection contre la conception de plus de 98% durant les six premiers mois.

References

1. **Vorherr, H.** The breast. Morphology, physiology and lactation. New York, Academic Press, 1974.
2. **Prentice, A. et al.** Cross-cultural differences in lactation performance. In: Hamosh, M. & Goldman, A., ed. Human lactation, 2: Maternal and environmental factors. New York, Plenum Press, 1986, p. 26.
3. **Saint, L. et al.** Yield and nutrient content of milk in eight women breast-feeding twins and one woman breast-feeding triplets. Br. j. nutr., **56**: 49–58 (1986).
4. **Helsing, E. & King, F.S.** Breast-feeding in practice. A manual for health workers. Oxford, Oxford University Press, 1982.
5. **Robinson, J.E. & Short, R.V.** Changes in breast sensitivity at puberty, during the menstrual cycle, and at parturition. Br. med. j., **1**: 1188–1191 (1977).
6. **Gunther, M.H.** Sore nipples: causes and prevention. Lancet, **2**: 590–592 (1945)
7. **Jelliffe, D.B. & Jelliffe, E.F.P.** Human milk in the modern world. Oxford, Oxford University Press, 1978.
8. **Hytten, F.** Weight gain in pregnancy. In: Hytten, F. &

Chamberlain, G., ed. *Clinical physiology in obstetrics*. Oxford, Blackwell Scientific Publications, 1980, p. 210.

9. **Hartmann, P.E. & Kent, J.C.** The subtlety of breast milk. *Breast-feeding review*, **13**: 14–18 (1988).

10. **Craig, R.K. & Campbell, P.N.** Molecular aspects of milk protein synthesis. In: Larson, B.L., ed. *Lactation, Vol. 4*. New York, Academic Press, 1978, p. 387.

11. **Kulski, J.K. & Hartmann, P.E.** Changes in milk composition during the initiation of lactation. *Aust. j. exp. biol. med. sci.*, **59** (1): 101–114 (1981).

12. **Prentice, A. et al.** Evidence for local feed-back control of human milk secretion. *Biochem. Soc. trans.*, **17**: 489–492 (1989).

13. **Cowie, A.T. et al.** Lactation. In: Heidelberg, G.F. et al., ed. *Hormonal control of lactation*. (Monographs in Endocrinology, Vol. 15). Berlin, Springer Verlag, 1980, pp. 1–275.

14. **Peaker, M. & Wild, C.J.** Milk secretion: autocrine control. *News in physiol. sciences*, **2**: 12406 (1987).

15. **Howie, P.W. et al.** The relationship between suckling-induced prolactin response and lactogenesis. *J. clin. endoc. metab.*, **50**: 670–673 (1980).

16. **Allen, L.H. et al.** Maternal factors affecting lactation. In: Hamosh, M. & Goldman, A.S., ed. *Human lactation, 2: Maternal and environmental factors*. New York, Plenum Press, 1986, p. 55.

17. **Chard, T.** The radioimmunoassay of oxytocin and vasopressin. *J. endocrinol.*, **58**: 143–160 (1973).

18. **Cobo, E.** Neuroendocrine control of milk ejection in women. In: Josimovich, J.B. et al., ed. *Lactogenic hormones, fetal nutrition and lactation*. New York, Wiley, 1974, p. 433.

19. **Beischer, N.A. et al.** *Care of the pregnant woman and her baby*. London, Saunders/Bailliere Tindall, 1989, p. 322.

20. **Lind, J. et al.** The effect of cry stimulus on the lactating breast of primiparas. In: Morris, N., ed. *Psychosomatic medicine in obstetrics and gynecology*. Third International Congress, London, 1971.

21. **Newton, N.** Psycho-social aspects of the mother/father/child unit. In: Hambreaus, L. & Sjölin, S., ed. *The mother/child dyad. Nutritional aspects* (Symposia of the Swedish Nutrition Foundation XIV). Stockholm, Almquist & Wiksell, 1979, p. 18.

22. **Barowicz, T.** Inhibitory effect of adrenaline on the oxytocin release in the ewe during the milk-ejection reflex. *J. dairy res.*, **46**: 41–46 (1979).

23. **Cooper, A.P.**, quoted in **Blanc, B.** Biochemical aspects of human milk: comparison with bovine milk. *Wld rev. nutr. diet.*, **36**: 1 (1981).

24. **Newton, M. & Newton, N.R.** The letdown reflex in human lactation. *J. pediatr.*, **33**: 698–704 (1948).

25. **Newton, N.** The role of oxytocin reflexes in the three inter-personal reproductive acts: coitus, birth and breast-feeding. In: Carenza, L. et al., ed. *Clinical psycho-endocrinology in reproduction*. (Proc. of the Serono Symposia, Vol. 22). New York, Academic Press, 1978, p. 411.

26. **Virden, S.F.** Relationship between infant-feeding method and maternal role adjustment. *J. nurs. midw.*, **33**: 31–35 (1988).

27. **Widstrom, A.M. et al.** Gastric suction in healthy newborn infants: effects on circulation and feeding behaviour. *Acta paediatr. Scand.*, **76**: 566–572 (1987).

28. **Woolridge, M.W.** The "anatomy" of infant sucking. *Midwifery*, **2**: 164–171 (1986).

29. **Meier, P. & Anderson, G.C.** Responses of small preterm infants to bottle- and breast-feeding. *Maternal and child nursing*, **12**: 97–105 (1987).

30. **Inch, S. & Garforth, S.** Establishing and maintaining breast-feeding. In: Chalmers, I. et al., ed. *Effective care in pregnancy and childbirth*. Oxford, Oxford University Press, 1989.

31. **Host, A. et al.** A prospective study of cow's milk allergy in exclusively breast-fed infants. Incidence, pathogenetic role of early inadvertent exposure to cows' milk formula, and characterization of bovine milk protein in human milk. *Acta paediatr. Scand.*, **77**: 663–670 (1988).

32. **Righard, L.** Les habitudes en salle d'accouchement et le succès de l'allaitement maternel. *Les dossiers de l'obstétrique*, **170**: 16–17 (1990).

33. **Royal College of Midwives.** *Successful breast-feeding: a handbook for midwives and others helping the breast-feeding mother*. London, 1988.

34. **Newton, N.** Nipple pain and nipple damage. *J. pediatr.*, **41**: 411–423 (1952).

35. **Minchin, M.K.** *Breastfeeding matters*. Sydney, Allen & Unwin, 1989, pp. 130–149.

36. **Hartmann, P.E. & Kulski, J.K.** Changes in the composition of the mammary secretion of women after abrupt termination of breast-feeding. *J. physiol.* **275**: 1–11 (1978).

37. **Egli, G.E. et al.** The influence of the number of feedings on milk production. *Pediatrics*, **27**: 314–317 (1961).

38. **Hartmann, P.E. & Prosser, C.G.** Physiological basis of longitudinal changes in human milk yield and composition. *Fed. Proc.*, **9**: 2448–2453 (1984).

39. **Wassenberger, J. et al.** Is there an excess of saturated fat in infant formula? *J. Am. Med. Assoc.*, **254**: 3047–3048 (1985).

40. *Quantity and quality of breast milk. Report on the WHO Collaborative Study on Breast-feeding*. Geneva, World Health Organization, 1985.

41. **Hibberd, C.M. et al.** Variation in the composition of breast milk during the first five weeks of lactation: implications for the feeding of pre-term infants. *Arch. dis. child.*, **57**: 658–662 (1982).

42. **Lönnerdal, B. et al.** Breast milk composition in Ethiopian and Swedish mothers. II. Lactose and protein contents. *Amer. j. clin. nutr.*, **29**: 1134–1141 (1976).

43. **Hambreaus, L. et al.** Nutritional aspects of breast milk versus cow's milk formula. In: Hambreaus, L. et al., ed. *Food and immunology*. Stockholm, Almquist & Wiksell, 1977, p. 116.

44. **Raiha, N.C.R. et al.** Milk-protein intake in the term infant. I. Metabolic responses and effects on growth. *Acta paediatr. Scand.*, **75**: 881–886 (1986).

45. **Raiha, N.C.R. et al.** Milk-protein intake in the term infant. II. Effects on amino acid concentrations. *Acta paediatr. Scand.*, **75**: 887–892 (1986).

46. **Gunther, M.** *Infant feeding*. London, Methuen, 1970.

47. **Raiha, N.C.** Nutritional proteins in milk and the protein requirement of normal infants. *Pediatrics*, **75**: 5142–5145 (1985) and **76**: 329 (1985) (letter).

48. **Cavagni, G. et al.** Passage of food antigens into the circulation of breast-fed infants with atopic dermatitis. *Ann. allergy*, **61**: 361–365 (1988).

49. **Cavell, B.** Gastric emptying in pre-term infants. *Acta paediatr. Scand.*, **68**: 725–730 (1979).

50. **Lawrence, R.A.** *Breast-feeding: a guide for the medical profession.* St. Louis, C.V. Mosby Co., 1989, p. 85.

51. **Hamosh, M. et al.** Lipids in milk and the first steps in their digestion. In: Current issues in feeding the normal infant. *Pediatrics*, **1**: 146–150 (1985) (Suppl. No. 75).

52. **Gaull, G.E. et al.** Milk protein quantity and quality in low-birth-weight infants. III. Effect on sulphur amino acids in the plasma and urine. *J. pediatr.*, **90**: 348–355 (1977).

53. **Atkinson, S.A. & Lönnerdal, B.** *Proteins and non-protein nitrogen in human milk.* CRC Press, 1989.

54. **Thompkinson, D.K. & Mathur, B.N.** Physiological response of neonates to lipids of human and bovine milk. *Austr. j. nutr. diet.*, **46**: 67–70 (1989).

55. **Crawford, M.A. et al.** Milk lipids and their variability. *Curr. med. res. opin.*, 4 (suppl. 1): 33–43 (1976).

56. **Bitman, J. et al.** Lipid composition of prepartum, preterm and term milk. In: Hamosh, M. & Goldman, A.S., ed. *Human lactation, 2: Maternal and environmental factors.* New York, Plenum Press, 1986.

57. **Lawrence, R.A.** reference 50, p. 73–77.

58. **Drewett, R.F.** Returning to the suckled breast: a further test of Hall's hypothesis. *Early hum. dev.*, **6**: 161–163 (1982).

59. **Woolridge, M.W. et al.** Individual patterns of milk intake during breast-feeding. *Early hum. dev.*, **7**: 265–272 (1982).

60. **Morley, R. et al.** Mother's choice to provide breast milk and developmental outcome. *Arch. dis. child.*, **63**: 1382–1385 (1988).

61. **Guthrie, H.A. et al.** Fatty acid patterns in human milk. *J. pediatr.*, **90**: 39–41 (1977).

62. **Clandinin, M.T. & Chappell, J.E.** Long-chain polyenoic essential fatty acids in human milk: Are they of benefit to the newborn? In: Schaub, J., ed. *Composition and physiological properties of human milk.* Amsterdam, Elsevier, 1985, pp. 213–224.

63. **Jackson, K.A. & Gibson, R.A.** A comparison of long-chain polyunsaturates in infant foods with breast milk. *Breast-feeding review*, **13**: 38–39 (1988).

64. **Gibson, R.A. & Kneebone, G.M.** Fatty acid composition of infant formulae. *Austr. paediatr. j.*, **17**: 46–53 (1981).

65. **Wales, J.K.H. et al.** Milk bolus obstruction secondary to the early introduction of premature baby milk formula: an old problem re-emerging in a new population. *Eur. j. paediatr.*, **148**: 676–678 (1989).

66. **Koletzko, B. et al.** Intestinal milk bolus obstruction in formula-fed premature infants given high doses of calcium. *J. pediatr. gastroent. nutr.*, **7**: 548–553; commentary 484–485 (1988).

67. **Robert, A.** Cytoprotection by prostaglandins. *Gastroenterol.*, **77**: 761–767 (1979).

68. **Chappell, J.E. et al.** Comparative prostaglandin content of human milk. In: Hamosh, M. & Goldman, A., ed. *Human lactation 2: Maternal and environmental factors.* New York, Plenum Press, 1986, pp. 175–186.

69. **Watkins, J.B.** Lipid digestion and absorption. In: Current issues in feeding the normal infant. *Pediatrics*, **1**: 151–156 (1985) (Suppl. No. 75).

70. **Freier, S. & Faber, J.** Loss of immune components during the processing of human milk. In: Williams, A.F. & Baum, J.D., ed. *Human milk banking.* New York, Raven Press, 1984, pp. 123–132.

71. **Hahn, P.** Obesity and atherosclerosis as a consequence of early weaning. In: Ballabriga, A., ed. *Weaning: why, what and when?* New York, Raven Press, 1987, pp. 93–113.

72. **Bullen, C.L.** Infant feeding and the faecal flora. In: Wilkinson, A.W. ed. *The immunology of infant feeding.* New York, Plenum Press, 1981, pp. 41–53.

73. **Bullen, C.L. & Willis, A.T.** Resistance of the breast-fed infant to gastroenteritis. *Br. med. j.*, **3**: 338–343 (1971).

74. **Woolridge, M.W. & Fisher, C.** 'Colic', overfeeding and symptoms of lactose malabsorption in the baby: a possible artefact of feed management. *Lancet*, **2**: 1382–1384 (1988).

75. **Moore, D.J. et al.** Breath-hydrogen response to milk containing lactose in colicky and non-colicky infants. *J. pediatr.*, **113**: 979–984 (1988).

76. **Gebre-Medhin, M. et al.** Breast-milk composition in Ethiopian and Swedish mothers. I. Vitamin A and beta-carotene. *Am. j. clin. nutr.*, **29**: 441–451 (1976).

77. **von Kries, R. et al.** Vitamin K deficiency in breast-fed infants. In: Goldman, A.S. et al. *Human lactation, 3: Effects on the recipient infant.* New York, Plenum Press, 1987. See also *Ped. res.*, **22**: 513–517 (1987).

78. **Greer F.R. et al.** Water-soluble vitamin D in human milk: a myth. *Pediatrics*, **69**: 238 (1982).

79. **Specker, B.L. et al.** Vitamin D. In: Tsang, R.C. & Nichols, B.L., ed. *Nutrition during infancy.* St. Louis, CV Mosby Co., 1988, p. 268.

80. **Rao, R.A. & Subrahmanyan, I.** An investigation on the thiamine content of mother's milk in relation to infantile convulsions. *Indian j. med. res.*, **52**: 1198 (1964).

81. **Ekstrand, J.** No evidence of transfer of fluoride from plasma to breast milk. *Br. med. j.*, **283**: 761–762 (1981).

82. **Saarinen, U.M. & Siimes, M.A.** Iron absorption from breast milk, cow's milk and iron-supplemented formula: an opportunistic use of changes in total body iron determined by hemoglobin, ferritin and body weight in 132 infants. *Pediatr. res.*, **13**: 143–147 (1979).

83. **Picciano, M.F.** Trace elements in human milk and infant formulas. In: Chandra, R.K., ed. *Trace elements in the nutrition of children.* New York, Raven Press, 1985, pp. 157–174.

84. **Oski, F.A. & Landow, S.A.** Inhibition of iron absorp-

tion from human milk by baby food. *Am. j. dis. child.*, **134**: 159–160 (1980).

85. **Oski, F.A.** Is bovine milk a health hazard? *Pediatrics*, **75** (part 2): 182–186 (1985).

86. **International Nutritional Anemia Consultative Group (INACG).** *Iron deficiency in women.* Washington, DC, The Nutrition Foundation, 1981.

87. **Simmer, K. et al.** Are iron folate supplements harmful? *Am. j. clin. nutr.*, **45**: 122–125 (1987).

88. **Fenton, V. et al.** Iron stores in pregnancy. *Br. j. haematol.*, **37**: 145–149 (1977).

89. **Rios, E. et al.** Relationship of maternal and infant iron stores as assessed by determination of plasma ferritin. *Pediatrics*, **55**: 694–699 (1975).

90. **Murray, M.J. et al.** The effect of iron status of Nigerian mothers and that of their infants at birth and six months, on concentration of Fe in breast milk. *Br. j. nutr.*, **39**: 627–630 (1978).

91. **Sturgeon, P.** Studies of iron requirements in infants. III. Influence of supplemental iron during normal pregnancy on mother and infant. B. The infant. *Br. j. haematol.*, **5**: 45–55 (1959).

92. **Sandstrom, B.** Zinc absorption from human milk, cow's milk and infant formulas. *Am. j. dis. child.*, **137**: 726–729 (1983).

93. **Mason, K.E.** A conspectus of research of copper metabolism and requirement in man. *J. nutr.*, **109**: 1981–2066 (1979).

94. **Wilson, J.F. et al.** Milk-induced gastrointestinal bleeding in infants with hypochromic microcytic anemia. *J. Am. Med. Assoc.*, **189**: 568–572 (1964).

95. **Smith, A.M. et al.** Selenium intakes and status of human milk and formula-fed infants. *Am. j. clin. nutr.*, **35**: 521–526 (1982).

96. **Smith, A.M. & Picciano, M.F.** Selenium nutrition during lactation and early infancy. In: Goldman, A.S. ed. *Human lactation, 3: The effects of human milk on the recipient infant.* New York, Plenum Press, 1987, pp. 81–87.

97. **Deelstra, H. et al.** Daily chromium intakes by infants in Belgium. *Acta paediatr. Scand.*, **77**: 402–407 (1988).

98. **Collipp, P.J. et al.** Aluminium contamination of infant formulas and learning disability. *Ann. nutr. metab.*, **27**: 488–494 (1983).

99. **Koo, W.W. et al.** Aluminium contamination of infant formulas. *J. parenter. enter. nutr.*, **12**: 170–173 (1988).

100. **Dabeka, R.W. & Mackenzie, A.D.** Lead and cadmium levels in commercial infant foods and dietary intake by infants 0–1 year old. *Food addit. contam.*, **5**: 333–342 (1988).

101. **Chisolm, J.J.** Pediatric exposures to lead, arsenic, cadmium, and methyl mercury. In: Chandra, R.K., ed. *Trace elements in nutrition of children.* New York, Raven Press, 1985, pp. 229–261.

102. **Chanoine, J.P. et al.** Increased recall rate at screening for congenital hypothyroidism in breast-fed infants born to iodine-overloaded mothers. *Arch. dis. child.*, **63**: 1207–1210 (1988).

103. *Minor and trace elements in breast milk. Report of a Joint WHO/IAEA Collaborative Study.* Geneva, World Health Organization, 1989.

104. **Hartmann, P.E. & Kent, J.C.** The subtlety of breast milk. *Breast-feeding review*, **13**: 14–18 (1988).

105. **Koldovsky, O. et al.** Hormones in milk: their presence and possible physiological significance. In: Goldman, A.S. et al., ed. *Human Lactation, 3: The effects of human milk on the recipient infant.* New York, Plenum Press, 1987, pp. 183–196.

106. **Aynsley-Green, A.** Hormones and postnatal adaptation to enteral nutrition. *J. pediatr. gastroent. nutr.*, **2**: 418–428 (1983).

107. **Morriss, F.H.** Growth factors in milk. In: Howell, R.R. et al., ed. *Human milk in infant nutrition and health.* Springfield, C.C. Thomas, 1986, pp. 98–114.

108. **Gaull, G.E. et al.** Significance of growth modulators in human milk. In: Current issues in feeding the normal infant. *Pediatrics* (Suppl.), **75**: 142–145 (1985).

109. **Werner, H. et al.** Growth hormone releasing factor and somatostatin concentrations in the milk of lactating women. *Eur. j. pediatr.*, **147**: 252–256 (1988).

110. **Björksten, B.** Does breast-feeding prevent the development of allergy? *Immunology today*, **4**: 215–217 (1983).

111. **Wilson, N.W. & Hamburger, R.N.** Allergy to cow's milk in the first year of life and its prevention. *Ann. allergy*, **61**: 323–326 (1988).

112. **Kajosaari, M. & Saarinen, U.M.** Prophylaxis of atopic disease by six months total solid food elimination. *Acta. pediatr. Scand.*, **72**: 411–414 (1983).

113. **Goldman, A.S. et al.** Anti-inflammatory properties of breast milk. *Acta paediatr. Scand.*, **75**: 689–695 (1986).

114. **Victora, C.G. et al.** Evidence for protection by breast-feeding against infant deaths from infectious diseases in Brazil. *Lancet*, **2**: 319–322 (1987).

115. **Behar, M.** The role of feeding and nutrition in the pathogeny and prevention of diarrheic processes. *Bull. Pan Am. Hlth Org.*, **9**: 1 (1975).

116. **Cunningham, A.S.** Breast-feeding, bottle-feeding and illness: an annotated bibliography 1986. In Jelliffe, D. & Jelliffe, E.F.P., ed. *Programmes to promote breastfeeding.* Oxford, Oxford University Press, 1988, pp. 448–480.

117. **Evensen, S.** *Relationship between infant morbidity and breast-feeding versus artificial feeding in industrialized countries: a review of literature.* Copenhagen, WHO Regional Office for Europe, 1983. (ICP/NUT/010/6).

118. **Saarinen, U.M.** Prolonged breast-feeding as prophylaxis for recurrent otitis media. *Acta paediatr. Scand.*, **71**: 567–571 (1982).

119. **Greco, L. et al.** Case-control study on nutritional risk factors in celiac disease. *J. pediatr. gastroent. nutr.*, **7**: 395–399 (1988).

120. **Koletzko, S. et al.** Role of infant-feeding practices in development of Crohn's disease in childhood. *Br. med. j.*, **298**: 1617–1618 (1989).

121. **Mayer, E.-J. et al.** Reduced risk of IDDM among breast-fed children: the Colorado IDDM registry. *Diabetes*, **37**: 1625–1632 (1988).

122. **Davis, M.K. et al.** Infant feeding and childhood cancer. *Lancet*, **2**: 365–368 (1988).

123. **Labbok, M.H. & Henderson, G.E.** Does breast-feeding protect against malocclusion? *Am. j. prev. med.*, **3**: 227–232 (1987).

124. **Smith, F.B.** *The people's health, 1830–1910*. Canberra, Australian National Press, 1979, p. 91.

125. **Renfrew, M.J.** *What we don't know about breast-feeding. Breast-feeding review*, **13**: 105–110 (1989).

126. **Howie, P.W.** Protective effect of breast-feeding against infection among infants in a Scottish city. *Br. med. j.*, **300**: 11–16 (1990)

127. **Walker, W.A.** Absorption of protein and protein fragments in the developing intestine: role of immunologic/allergic reactions. In: Current issues in feeding the normal infant. *Pediatrics (Suppl.)*, **75**: 167–171 (1985).

128. **Hanson, L.A. et al.** Breast-feeding protects against infection and allergy. *Breast-feeding review*, **13**: 19–22 (1988).

129. **Ogra, P.L. et al.** Immunology of breast milk: maternal and neonatal interactions. In: Freier, S. & Eidelman, A.I. *Human milk. Its biological and social value.* Amsterdam, Excerpta Medica, 1980, p. 115.

130. **Hanson, L.A. et al.** Protective factors in milk and the development of the immune system. In: Current Issues in feeding the normal infant. *Pediatrics (Suppl.)*, **75**: 172–176 (1985).

131. **Brandtzaeg, P.** The secretory immune system of lactating human mammary glands compared with other exocrine organs. In: Ogra, P.L. & Dayton, D.H., ed. *Immunology of breast milk*. New York, Raven Press, 1979, p. 99.

132. **Prentice, A.** Breast-feeding increases concentration of IgA in infants' urine. *Arch. dis. child.*, **62**: 792–795 (1987).

133. **Goldblum, R.M. et al.** Human milk enhances the urinary secretion of immunologic factors in LBW infants. *Pediatr. res.*, **25**: 184–188 (1989).

134. **Usowicz, A.G. et al.** Does gastric acid protect the preterm infant from bacteria in unheated human milk? *Early hum. dev.*, **16**: 27–33 (1988).

135. **Carrion, V. & Egan, E.** Gastric pH and quantitative bacterial colonization of the stomach in infants < 2500 g. *Ped. res.*, **23** (4, pt. 2): 481A (1988).

136. **Raiha, N.** In: Kretchmer, N. & Minkowski, A., ed. *Nutritional adaptation of the gastrointestinal tract of the newborn.* New York, Raven Press, 1983, p. 163.

137. **May, J.T.** Microbial contaminants and antimicrobial properties of human milk. *Microbiol. sci.*, **5**: 42–46 (1988).

138. **Duffy, L.C. et al.** The effects of breast-feeding on rotavirus induced gastroenteritis: a prospective study. *Am. j. publ. hlth*, **76**: 259–263 (1986).

139. **Gendrel, D. et al.** Giardiasis and breast-feeding in urban Africa. *Ped. infect. dis. j.*, **8**: 58–59 (1989).

140. **Gillin, F.D. et al.** Human milk kills parasitic intestinal protozoa. *Science*, **221**: 1290–1292 (1983).

141. **Butte, N.F. et al.** Human milk intake and growth in exclusively breast-fed infants. *J. pediatr.*, **104**: 187–195 (1984).

142. **Montandon, C.M.** Formula intake of one- and four-month-old infants. *J. pediatr. gastroent. nutr.*, **5**: 434–438 (1986).

143. **Prentice, A.M. & Prentice, A.** Energy costs of lactation. *Ann. rev. nutr.*, **8**: 63–79 (1988).

144. **Jensen, R.G. & Neville, M.** *Human lactation: milk components and methodologies.* New York, Plenum Press, 1985.

145. **Uvnäs-Moberg, K.** The gastrointestinal tract in growth and reproduction. *Scientific American*, **255**: 60–65 (1989).

146. WHO Technical Report Series No. 724, 1985 (*Energy and protein requirements*: report of a Joint FAO/WHO/UNU Expert Consultation), Ch. 6, pp. 71–112.

147. **Dusdieker, L.B. et al.** Effect of supplemental fluid on human milk production. *J. pediatr.*, **106**: 207–211 (1985).

148. **Short, R.V.** Breast-feeding. *Scientific American*, **250**: 23–29 (1984).

149. Consensus Statement. Breast-feeding as a family planning method. *Lancet*, **2**: 1204–1205 (1988).

3. Health factors which may interfere with breast-feeding

Breast-feeding is the feeding method of choice for all normal infants because of its many advantages for the health of infants and mothers alike. There are, however, a number of situations—fortunately relatively infrequent—where infants cannot, or should not, be breast-fed. Such circumstances can be related to the health of infants or mothers; in either case, breast-milk substitutes may be needed for extended periods. In this context, it is useful to distinguish between infants who should not receive breast milk at all and infants who cannot be fed at the breast, but for whom breast milk is still the food of choice. There is also a tiny minority of infants who should not be fed either on breast milk or any milk-based substitute; special preparations are required in such cases. Finally, there are also a number of situations which are frequently thought to be an impediment to breast-feeding but which in fact generally are not; these, too, are discussed.

Introduction

Adequate diet is more critical in early infancy than at any other time in life. This is because of the infant's high nutritional requirements in relation to body weight (see chapter 4) and the influence of proper or faulty nutrition during the first months on future health and development. Moreover, the infant is more sensitive to abnormal nutritional situations and less adaptable than in later life to different types, forms, proportions and quantities of food.

As noted earlier, breast-feeding is an unequalled way of providing ideal food for the healthy growth and development of all normal infants. In addition, as discussed in chapters 2 and 6, the anti-infective properties of breast milk help to protect infants against disease and there is an important relation between breast-feeding and child-spacing. There are, however, a number of health situations—fortunately infrequent—where infants cannot, or should not, be breast-fed, and where alternative sources of safe and adequate nutrition must be found. This chapter discusses situations where breast-feeding is not possible, or is contraindicated, for reasons related to the physical health of the infant or the mother, and where breast-milk substitutes may therefore be needed for extended periods. Other situations, including the exercise of choice with regard to infant-feeding mode, are not reviewed here.

First it is useful to distinguish between infants who should not receive breast milk at all and infants who cannot be fed at the breast, but for whom breast milk is still the food of choice. There is also a tiny minority of infants who should not be fed either on breast milk or any milk-based substitute, and for whom special preparations are required. Finally, there are a number of situations which are frequently thought to be an impediment to breast-feeding but

which in fact generally are not; these also will be considered here. Low-birth-weight infants, who have special nutritional requirements arising from their rapid growth rate and developmental immaturity, are dealt with in chapter 5.

Possible contraindications to breast-feeding

Situations related to infant health

Inborn errors of metabolism. Some congenital and hereditary metabolic disorders, characterized by specific enzyme deficiencies, severely limit or render impossible the use of certain milk components. Serious health disturbances may result unless dietary intake of the components in question is restricted or, in some cases, completely eliminated. Some of these disorders, such as congenital adrenal hyperplasia or propionic acidaemia, are usually only apparent as mild failure to thrive until the infant is weaned and the symptoms abruptly worsen (1). Others are actually alleviated by breast-feeding (2). There are three metabolic disorders of particular interest in this context: galactosaemia, phenylketonuria and maple-syrup urine disease.

Galactosaemia. There are two main forms of this disease; one is characterized by a deficiency of galactokinase, which is an enzyme required for the breakdown of galactose, a component of lactose. If infants who have this disease are fed breast milk, or any lactose-containing preparation, their galactose blood level rises, sugar appears in the urine and clinically they develop cataracts.

The other form of the disease is even more serious. It is due to a deficiency of another enzyme, galactose-

1-phosphate uridyl transferase, which is required later in the metabolism of galactose. The resulting metabolite accumulating in the blood produces even greater damage than the first form of the disease. Symptoms in the infant include diarrhoea, vomiting, hepatomegaly, jaundice and splenomegaly. If lactose is not eliminated from the diet, cataracts, hepatic cirrhosis and mental retardation result.

If there is reason to suspect galactosaemia, it can be diagnosed through laboratory tests, either during the intrauterine period or immediately following birth. Since lactose must be eliminated from the diet of infants suffering from both forms of the disease, they cannot be fed either on human or other milk, including the usual breast-milk substitutes. Specially formulated milk-based, but lactose-free, preparations, or soya-based formulas are required. Some infants have benefited from the use of lactose-hydrolysed human milk (3). Fortunately, this disease is rare; prevalence figures are available only from industrialized countries where they vary between 1 in 20 000 and 1 in 200 000 infants (0.5–5 per 100 000 population) (4).

Phenylketonuria. This condition is characterized by defective metabolism of the amino acid phenylalanine. It is due to absence in the liver of the enzyme phenylalanine hydroxylase, and its most serious clinical manifestation is moderate-to-severe mental retardation. Diagnosis can be made soon after birth by laboratory tests, which are performed routinely in many countries. The development of the clinical manifestations of this condition can be avoided by providing a low-phenylalanine diet. Fortunately, breast milk contains a low concentration of this amino acid, much lower in fact than cow's milk. Thus infants suffering from phenylketonuria may be breast-fed while their phenylalanine blood levels are monitored. Breast milk should be supplemented with or replaced by a special low-phenylalanine formula if concentrations reach dangerous levels (5, 6). Prevalence figures from industrialized countries vary between 1 in 5000 and 1 in 100 000 infants (1–20 per 100 000 population) (7).

Maple-syrup urine disease. This disease is due to a defect in the metabolism of the branched-chain amino acids valine, leucine and isoleucine, which are normal components of all natural proteins. The specific enzymatic deficiency is not yet well identified. It is characterized by the urine's typical maple-syrup odour, refusal of food, vomiting, metabolic acidosis and progressive neurological and mental deterioration. Special synthetic formulas, low in the non-tolerated amino acids, have been developed for the feeding of such infants, although outcomes are frequently poor (8). As in the case of phenylketonuria, breast milk can be combined with these products and partial breast-feeding may therefore be possible (6). The disease, which is fatal within the first months of life unless treated, is very rare with a prevalence of only about 1 in 200 000 infants (0.5 per 100 000 population) (9).

Cleft lip and cleft palate. Infants born with a cleft lip or cleft palate may have difficulty creating the negative pressure necessary for breast-feeding, or in stripping the milk from the breast by compression of the teat against the palate (see chapter 2). The seriousness of the problem depends on the extent of the lesion and the protractility of the breast. Most infants with a cleft lip but intact palate manage to feed, and their mothers soon learn to help them by closing with their breast the opening between mouth and nose; the protractility of breast tissue determines the extent to which this is possible. For such infants breast-feeding may in fact be easier than bottle-feeding. The breast, after all, actively ejects milk (see chapter 2), and the mother can express it as the child feeds. In contrast, much greater effort is needed to extract milk from a bottle, unless the teat hole is very large or the milk is squeezed out of a specially designed bottle. However, delivering an antigenic breast-milk substitute in this way poses some risks if aspiration should occur.

As with cleft lip, the possibility of breast-feeding in cases of cleft palate depends on how extensive the defect is. If it is unilateral and small, the mother may be able to place her breast in a way that makes feeding possible. Still, feeding may not be efficient enough, in which case milk production could diminish. Under such circumstances letting the infant suck at the breast and then expressing the milk manually will satisfy the infant's nutritional needs while helping to maintain lactation performance.

In cases of very extensive bilateral malformation, feeding from either a natural or artificial teat may be impossible, and a spoon, small cup, syringe or similar device will have to be used. Temporary palatal obturators can be devised, which help the infant to feed. A supplemental feeding system may also be of use; this consists of a fine tube, placed beside the nipple, which delivers previously expressed breast milk to the infant while at the breast.

The problem posed by cleft palate is less one of having to choose between breast milk or a breast-milk substitute than having to overcome an infant's inability to feed. The food of choice for such infants remains breast milk, both because of its nutritional and immunological advantages and the importance of maintaining lactation so that they can be breast-fed normally once the defect has been corrected. In fact, the high incidence of otitis media and speech defect in these children suggests that it would be preferable for them to receive only breast milk, and thus avoid the antigenic proteins and the oro-facial activity of artificial feeding, as far as is possible. Better outcomes are documented in breast-fed than in artificially fed infants (10). The incidence of cleft lip is on the order of 1 per 1000 infants, while that for cleft palate is 1 in 2500 infants (respectively, 1 and 0.4 per 1000 population) (11).

Situations related to maternal health

Lactation failure. Lactation failure means the inability of a woman to produce significant amounts of milk after giving birth, and should be distinguished from "perceived milk insufficiency", which is discussed later. Lactation failure is one of the reasons frequently given by mothers for not breast-feeding their infants; it is claimed to occur almost exclusively in industrialized countries and in the higher socioeconomic groups in urban areas of developing countries. Yet the women in question are, in the main, healthy and well-nourished, with healthy and strong infants, and there is no apparent physiological reason for their not being able to secrete milk.

In contrast, in traditional societies, even women who live in unsanitary conditions, who are poorly nourished and often ill, who engage in strenuous physical labour, and who bear the greatest number of low-birth-weight infants do not generally fail to secrete milk. For example, in the WHO collaborative study on breast-feeding (12), it was found that out of a total of 3898 mothers studied in Nigeria and Zaire, not one was unable to secrete milk. This sample included both women from among the urban elite and those from poor urban and rural populations. In a prospective study undertaken in a small, poor Indian village in the mountains of Guatemala (13), children born during an 8-year period were followed longitudinally. All 448 infants born alive during the period, and who survived for 48 hours, were successfully breast-fed.

The incidence of lactation failure as a primary physiopathological phenomenon is not easily ascertained since it depends on being able to assess the proportion of women who, with no external influences that may interfere with lactation, are unable to secrete milk. Lactation performance is very sensitive both to early supplementation and to psychosocial factors that are frequently difficult to identify (see chapter 2 for a discussion of inhibition of the oxytocin reflex).

In industrialized countries the inability to lactate is closely associated with women who have little or no information about breast-feeding; have little or no experience with its mechanics; lack confidence about their ability to breast-feed; and have no close family member, friend or other means of social support to aid them in overcoming problems they may encounter in initiating breast-feeding. At the same time, these women are frequently exposed to a variety of social, economic and cultural influences that can be inimical to breast-feeding. Coincidentally or not, most also give birth in hospitals where attitudes and practices conducive to the suppression of lactation remain common (14, 15) (see Annex 1).

In contrast, in societies where breast-feeding is regarded as a natural physiological function and the only way to nourish an infant, and where it is highly valued and therefore strongly encouraged and supported by society in general and families in particular, lactation failure is virtually unknown. Women in these societies are also less often exposed to health systems likely to undermine lactation.

Based on limited clinical experience in industrialized countries, it appears that a maximum in the range of 1–5% of women experience lactation failure on purely physiological grounds (16). Observations made in traditional societies suggest an even lower figure. No attempt has yet been made to explain this discrepancy, as there has been no published research into possible etiologies.

Maternal illness. It is remarkable how reliably lactation continues despite many maternal health problems. Breast-feeding is contraindicated only in cases of severe maternal illness, e.g., heart failure or serious kidney, liver or lung disease. In rare cases of psychosis or severe postnatal depression, where an infant's life may be in danger if cared for by a disturbed mother, the necessary separation of mother and infant makes breast-feeding difficult. However, in current methods of caring for depressed women it is suggested that mother and infant should not be totally separated. Provided that drugs in use are not incompatible with lactation (see below), and that the mother wishes to breast-feed, there is no reason to wean such an infant, although feeding, like other contact, will have to be supervised. It can be important for her recovery that she should not feel that she has failed in this area as in others (17).

Most common illnesses in mothers are not in themselves reasons not to breast-feed. However, the possible transmission of infections to the infant merits more detailed consideration.

Mastitis. Breast inflammation is characterized by swelling, pain, redness and fever, but the inflammation is not necessarily infectious in origin (18). It occurs most frequently during the first weeks of lactation, and whenever more milk is being produced than is removed. The non-infectious causes of obstructive mastitis are reviewed elsewhere (19). One non-epidemic form of puerperal mastitis is a cellulitis of the interlobular connective tissue of the breast, usually produced by *Staphylococcus aureus*. The microorganisms found in breast milk during this type of infection are the same as those frequently found in the milk of non-infected mothers, that is, the common microorganisms of the mother's skin and mouth, which she shares with her infant from a few hours after birth with no negative consequences.

It has been suggested that early infection of the infant with this type of non-pathogenic microorganism plays an important role in building up the infant's defence mechanisms (*20*). Breast-feeding does not have to be interrupted during this type of mastitis; on the contrary, drainage of the breast is essential and it has been observed that the inflammation is of shorter duration and is less frequently complicated with abscesses when breast-feeding is continued (*21, 22*). If breast-feeding at the affected breast is too painful, milk should be expressed manually or with a pump, or by the vacuum produced when a heated glass jar is applied to the breast and allowed to cool. This usually causes symptoms to disappear within 36–48 hours, although treatment with antibiotics may be required in severe cases.

There is also an epidemic form of mastitis, which is a hospital-acquired infection due to pathogenic microorganisms. By the time symptoms are observed, both mother and infant have already been infected. Therapy is required for both, but, once again, breast-feeding should continue. Weaning would deprive the already infected infant of the many anti-microbial factors in breast milk, and substitute feeds encourage the growth of gut pathogens. Neither is desirable for an infant already exposed to risk.

Breast abscess. Breast abscess is a possible complication of mastitis, and is most likely whenever breast-feeding is abruptly interrupted (*21, 22*). Feeding should continue at the non-infected breast, and milk from the infected one gently expressed until it can once again be taken directly by the infant.

Urinary-tract infection. This is a commonly observed postpartum bacterial infection. Its treatment presents no problem for the infant, and breast-feeding should therefore continue.

Tuberculosis. Active tuberculosis should be investigated and treated during pregnancy, thus eliminating the danger of infecting the infant after birth. For this same reason, contacts should also be investigated and treated as required. Where an infective bacteriologically positive mother is discovered only after delivery, there is a danger of infecting the infant, not by breast-feeding as such, but rather as a result of close contact, both of which are otherwise beneficial. Under such circumstances, a mother should be treated, preferably with a short-course regimen of at least three drugs for the first 2 months of treatment (*23*); she becomes non-infective shortly

thereafter. Meanwhile her infant should receive a prophylactic dose of isoniazid for 6–12 months (10 mg per kg of body weight in a single daily dose) (*24*). It is also recommended that the infant receive BCG vaccine (*23*). Breast-feeding is all the more important since tuberculosis in a mother, which is diagnosed only after delivery, occurs most often among the lowest socioeconomic groups living in poor environmental conditions. Under such circumstances, not breast-feeding an infant only represents an additional unnecessary risk. Moreover, from the purely practical standpoint of limited living space, it may be quite impossible to separate mother and infant.

Viral infections. Common viral diseases like rubella, chicken pox, measles and mumps, though rare, can be observed in lactating mothers. Mumps can cause an extremely painful mastitis, for which there is no remedy but continued breast-feeding and time (*25*). In these situations, by the time of diagnosis the infant has alrady had every chance of being infected or immunized. There is, therefore, no reason to isolate the infant or to interrupt breast-feeding. On the contrary, breast milk's specific anti-infective properties serve to protect the infant who, although infected, will frequently not develop the disease itself.

There are a number of other viral infections, which also merit brief discussion.

● *Cytomegalovirus.* Intrauterine infection with cytomegalovirus (CMV) is a common cause of congenital anomalies. The infection is not dangerous for the infant after birth, however. A high proportion of healthy mothers (14% in one study in the USA) have CMV in their cervical secretions. Their infants become infected during delivery but do not develop any pathology (*26*). Similarly, CMV (and a specific antibody to CMV) will be excreted by the mother in breast milk or saliva with the inevitable result of infecting the infant, but again without adverse consequences (*27, 28*). Discovery of CMV in a lactating mother is thus no reason for discontinuing breast-feeding; on the contrary, breast-feeding is regarded as a primary form of immunization against such viral disease. While artificially fed infants may be infected less frequently than those who are breast-fed, they suffer more serious consequences (*29*).

● *Herpes simplex.* The infection of the neonate with human (alpha) herpes virus 1 or 2, resulting in a severe disease, occurs during passage through the birth canal of a mother who has active genital herpes lesions. Caesarean section is indicated if the lesions are detected in time, that is at the onset of labour (*30*). Breast milk is not infective under such circumstances and there is thus no reason for not breast-feeding. Careful hygienic handling of the infant is in any case required to prevent infection spreading from the mother's hands, mouth or clothing. Partners should avoid mouth-breast contact during periods of active oral herpes lesions. Lesions that develop on the breast should be covered during breast-feeding.

● *Hepatitis B.* The possibility of transmitting hepatitis B virus from an active infected or carrier mother to her neonate via breast-feeding cannot be excluded. In such a situation, however, the infant has already been exposed to a greater risk of infection through maternal blood, amniotic fluid and vaginal secretions during birth (*31*). Furthermore, in areas of high endemicity where there is a high prevalence of healthy carriers of the virus, environmental exposure is so frequent that the avoiding of breast-feeding provides very little protection while exposing the infant to a greater risk of other infections (*32*). Studies in England, where the prevalence of hepatitis B carriers is low, demonstrate that breast-feeding does not increase the rate of infection among infants (*32*). In the USA, where the prevalence of carriers is less than 1% overall, the American Academy of Pediatrics recommends the administration of hepatitis B immune globulin to infants of carrier mothers who breast-feed (*33*). Thus, in view of breast milk's numerous advantages and the fact that the risk of transmitting hepatitis B virus in this manner is negligible, active infected or carrier mothers in most parts of the world should be encouraged to breast-feed. Their infants should receive only breast milk. One study reports that hepatitis B antigen clearance was many times greater in infants who were only breast-fed (*34*).

● *Human immunodeficiency virus (HIV).* Human immunodeficiency virus has been cultured from the breast milk of HIV-infected mothers (*35*). In addition, there have been several case reports of infants acquiring HIV from mothers who first became infected from a blood transfusion shortly after delivery and then proceeded to breast-fed (*36, 37*). This may be because immediately after a mother first becomes infected with the virus there are high concentrations of virus but no antibody in her blood. However, among women who are already infected with HIV, the additional risk, *if any*, of HIV transmission from HIV-infected mothers through breast-feeding is considered to be very low.

In June 1987, WHO organized a technical consultation to review available information on the possible relationship between breast-feeding/breast milk and HIV transmission, and to identify further research needs in this area. The consultation's recommendations, which were reviewed and endorsed in the light of current information by a meeting of experts in December 1989, can be summarized as follows (*38*).

Breast-feeding should continue to be promoted, supported and protected in both developing and developed countries in view of the overall benefits of this infant-feeding method (see chapter 2). Breast milk may also be important in preventing intercurrent infections, which could accelerate progression of HIV-related disease in already infected infants. However, additional epidemiological and laboratory research is needed on the risks of HIV transmission through breast milk and on the potential benefits of breast milk in situations where infants have been exposed to HIV or are already infected.

If, for whatever reason, the biological mother cannot breast-feed or her milk is not available, and the use of pooled milk is considered, the report of isolation of HIV in breast milk should be taken into account. Pasteurization at 56°C for 30 minutes has been reported to inactivate the virus. Further research on the effectiveness of different methods of pasteurization is needed, however. As an additional precaution, the possibility of screening donors (in accordance with relevant WHO criteria (*39*)) should be considered, especially in areas where the prevalence of HIV infection is known to be high. Similarly, if, for whatever reason, the biological mother cannot breast-feed, or her milk is not available, and where wet-nursing is the next obvious choice, care may need to be taken in selecting the wet-nurse, bearing in mind her possible HIV infection status and that of the infant who is to be fed.

In individual situations where the mother is considered to be HIV-infected, and recognizing the difficulties inherent in assessing the infection status of the newborn, the known and potential benefits of breast-feeding should be compared with the theoretical, but apparently small, incremental risk to the infant of becoming infected through breast-feeding. Consideration should be given to the socio-economic and ecological environment of the mother–child pair and the extent to which alternatives can safely and effectively be used. In many circumstances, particularly where the safe and effective use of alternatives is not possible, breast-feeding by the biological mother should continue to be the feeding method of choice, irrespective of her HIV infection status.

Situations normally not a contraindication

Conditions related to the infant

Multiple births. The breast-feeding of twins presents no problem for a healthy, well-nourished mother as far as quantity of breast milk is concerned (*40*). A lactating mother's capacity for milk production is almost always greater than her actual production. Since secretion is determined to a large extent by demand, vigorous feeding by twins would stimulate lactation performance and permit a mother to produce enough milk to feed both. This result has been commonly observed where wet-nursing is concerned.

If the infants' birth weights are too low (< 1200 g), or their feeding ability is poor, breast milk may initially have to be expressed for manual feeding, in order to maintain lactation performance until the infants are able to take the breast directly (see chapters 2 and 5). Not all chronically malnourished mothers have the capacity to feed two infants adequately, although even marginally nourished Gambian women successfully breast-fed all the twins born to them (41, 42). Occasionally, supplementary feeding may also be necessary for the infants while breast-feeding is maintained.

There are many reports of mothers successfully breast-feeding triplets. Not infrequently, however, such infants' birth weights are low and their feeding ability is poor; thus, additional ways of supplying the mother's milk may also be required. The amounts involved are usually small while the infants are tiny and weak, and mothers can produce this volume with appropriate assistance. There is a tendency for milk volume to decline if mothers do not express frequently (5–6 times per day and once during the night) in the early weeks (43). A suitably designed breast-milk pump can be an invaluable aid in some cases.

Breast-feeding jaundice. In addition to the common jaundice of the newborn, which is not a reason for supplementation (44), there is a rare type of jaundice associated with breast-feeding that develops when the infant is about one week old (45). It lasts about two months and is characterized by high levels of unconjugated bilirubin in the blood. Abnormal bilirubin metabolism is associated with ingestion of the mature breast milk (though not the colostrum) of some mothers, though the specific responsible mechanism has yet to be identified. This is not necessarily harmful; recent research indicates that bilirubin may be an anti-oxidant of physiological importance to the neonate (46). Apart from jaundice the infant is generally healthy and develops normally; since the jaundice is temporary and produces no ill effects there is no reason to discontinue breast-feeding. It is in any case important to establish a differential diagnosis in order to eliminate other possible causes, which may have more serious consequences.

A positive diagnosis can be obtained by withholding the breast for 24–36 hours. A rapid and marked drop in bilirubin blood levels in the infant is observed, followed by a rise to lower-than-previous levels when breast-feeding is resumed. While conducting this test, lactation should be maintained by expressing milk. A brief interruption of breast-feeding (24–48 hours) may be necessary if bilirubin blood levels rise above 15 mg per 100 ml (256 μmol/l) (47). Breast-feeding can safely continue thereafter.

Haemorrhagic disease of the newborn. The vitamin K-dependent blood coagulation factors are low in normal full-term infants, and lower still in pre-term infants (see chapter 5). There is a further decrease in these factors by the second or third day after birth, with a gradual return to birth values by the seventh to tenth day of life. This condition is associated with a prolonged prothrombin time and blood coagulation time. The physiological significance of this progression for the infant is unknown. Vitamin K levels in breast milk depend on maternal intake in the last stage of pregnancy (48). Because colostrum and hindmilk have especially high concentrations of vitamin K, infants should be breast-fed without restriction from birth.

Although rarely observed in full-term infants, the transient deficiency of vitamin K-dependent factors is occasionally severe or prolonged in pre-term infants and results in gastrointestinal, nasal and intracranial bleeding, or bleeding following circumcision. The syndrome is not observed in artificially fed infants in whom the normal intestinal flora of the breast-fed infant, predominantly acidophilic, are replaced by alkaline flora having an abundance of *Escherichia coli* and a large proportion of anaerobic bacteria. Under these circumstances, vitamin K is synthesized in the intestinal lumen and its absorption corrects the coagulation defect. Even when vitamin K deficiency is severe, however, the condition is easily corrected by the intramuscular injection of a single 0.5–1 mg dose of vitamin K or 1–2 mg orally (49), and should thus not be considered a cause for discontinuing breast-feeding.

Diarrhoea. Diarrhoea is often wrongly diagnosed in the breast-fed infant by health workers unaware of the wide range of normal stool frequency and fluidity in healthy breast-fed infants, particularly in the first weeks. Excessive stool frequency and volume can result from poorly managed breast-feeding (see chapter 2). Although diarrhoea is much less common among breast-fed than bottle-fed infants, it does occur. There is no reason to stop, even temporarily, breast-feeding of an infant who has diarrhoea. On the contrary, infants who continue to breast-feed use a considerable proportion of ingested nutrients and generally fare better than infants who are denied nourishment and the many antimicrobial and therapeutic factors of breast milk. Breast milk substitutes would not be desirable under such circumstances; indeed, it is frequently their use that has caused the diarrhoea in the first place. Chapter 6 provides a detailed review of the infant and young child during periods of acute infection.

Conditions related to the mother

Breast cancer. Some epidemiological evidence suggests that, when other variables are controlled for, premenopausal breast cancer is less frequent among women who have lactated than among those who have not (51). For example, recent studies in the USA suggest that breast-feeding can nearly halve the risk of breast cancer relative to that of a parous woman who bottle-feeds her children; the longer a woman breast-feeds, the greater the protection (52, 53).

In any case, pregnancy and lactation do not present any additional risk if a mother develops breast cancer at the same time. Breast cancer which has been treated by surgery may be a reason to avoid pregnancy; if such a woman becomes pregnant, breast-feeding may be permitted depending on the general health of the mother and the adequacy of breast function. Some years ago, virus particles resembling those associated with breast cancer in mice were found in human milk. It was at one time thought that it could be possible for mothers to transmit the disease potential to their breast-fed daughters but epidemiological evidence has disproved this hypothesis (54).

Inverted nipples. Inverted nipples are a relatively rare physical malformation; mild cases can be treated at the antenatal clinic, although surgery may be required for more serious cases. For the majority of women so affected, however, breast-feeding is entirely possible, depending on the protractility of the breast tissue which changes under the influence of hormones during pregnancy and infant feeding (see chapter 2). Simple exercises a mother can perform during the last trimester of pregnancy may help prepare her nipples for successful breast-feeding (55–57).

Drug therapy. A lactating mother's need for drug treatment (58, 59) can sometimes cause difficulty. While nearly all drugs are secreted in breast milk, their concentration and possible effects on the breast-feeding infant vary considerably. Drug concentration in breast milk depends on the characteristics and pharmacokinetics of the drug itself (58) and the properties of human milk. The information available on many drugs is insufficient to make an appropriate judgement, and the continual arrival of new ones on the market poses additional problems. In general, the drug concentration in breast milk is very close to that in maternal plasma, and thus the quantity of drug ingested by the infant is a function of the amount of

milk consumed (60). The total ingested drug dose, however, is not sufficient by itself to judge the possibility of ill effects.

Some drugs, although present in breast milk, are not absorbed by the infant. On the other hand, the infant may react idiosyncratically to minute amounts of others. Drugs can also accumulate in neonates owing to their reduced clearance capabilities, or infants may have a specific sensitivity to drugs that are not particularly toxic for older children and adults. Thus, while most common drugs can be safely given to lactating mothers without causing significant risk to breast-fed infants, extreme caution must always be exercised (60). What follows are a number of general recommendations in this regard.

Drug therapy should be avoided in lactating mothers wherever possible. When drugs are indicated, those least likely to have negative repercussions on the infant should be selected first. Lactating women should preferably take drugs during or immediately after breast-feeding to avoid the period of maximum concentration in the blood (and milk). Where there is a strong indication for a drug that is known to be harmful to the breast-fed infant, breast-feeding should be temporarily interrupted while lactation is maintained.

The decision about using new drugs is more difficult when little or no information is available on possible ill effects for infants, and interruption of breast-feeding would normally be the safest course. However, when bottle-feeding itself places an infant at greater risk under given circumstances, it may be preferable to continue breast-feeding while monitoring the infant to detect possible undesirable effects. In any event, should the breast-fed infant of a mother who is taking drugs present symptoms that cannot be clearly accounted for by other means, the possibility of their being related to the drug in question should be thoroughly investigated.

The Committee on Drugs of the American Academy of Pediatrics has undertaken an extensive review of the literature and published a list (61) that includes:
— drugs that are contraindicated during breast-feeding such as amethopterin, ergotamine, gold salts and thiouracil, which are known to have harmful consequences for the infant;
— drugs that call for a temporary interruption of breast-feeding, for example any preparation resulting in radioactivity in breast milk for a variable period during which breast-feeding would not be advisable;
— drugs that are usually compatible with breast-feeding, among which are the large majority of the most commonly used preparations.

The most thorough and extensive overview ever

prepared of the effects of drugs on the breast-feeding mother and her child was published in 1988 following a 3-year study by the World Health Organization's Regional Office for Europe (60). All of the original evidence on which current knowledge is based has been re-examined. By rejecting so-called evidence that does not stand up to critical appraisal, the review provides a clear picture of what is known and, equally important, of what is still not known about drugs in breast milk and the effect of these substances on lactation and the infant. Much of the material is very reassuring; the real risks and uncertainties have been defined in such a way that they can be avoided. The review provides the basis for a critical re-assessment of lists prepared to guide health workers about the use of drugs during pregnancy and lactation.

The use of hormonal contraceptives by lactating women presents a number of special problems (62). Products containing estrogen frequently cause a significant drop in the amount of breast milk secreted, while products containing progestogen have been found to reduce the fat concentration in breast milk. These steroids will also be present in breast milk. The amounts actually ingested by the infant in such cases are very low, although the amount of steroid transferred appears to be greater in the case of the progestogen-only pill (63). However, the synthetic steroids normally used in contraceptive pills are not as rapidly metabolized as naturally occurring ones and can cause breast engorgement and other secondary sex changes in the infant.

Contraception is generally not required during the first months of lactation owing to lactational amenorrhoea and anovulation in mothers whose infants are fed exclusively and frequently on breast milk (64). When full protection is desired, or when there is doubt about the timing of the initiation of ovulation, non-hormonal contraceptive methods should be employed. If hormonal methods must be used, preference should be given to products containing only progestogen. (See also, in chapter 1, the discussion on the effect of anaesthetic or drugs on the infant.)

Environmental pollutants. Undesirable chemical compounds may be found in breast milk as a result of environmental contamination. Most readily monitored, though not necessarily the most toxic, are the chlorinated insecticides, especially dichlorodiphenol trichloroethane (DDT) and similar compounds, because of their high level of toxicity. DDT is a fat-soluble chemical that is biologically non-degradable; it accumulates in the fat tissues of animals that are exposed to it. The only significant way in which the product can be excreted is via breast milk, where it concentrates in the fat component.

DDT has been found in human milk in many places in the world. Particularly high concentrations have been observed in areas where DDT has been widely used, without any control, in the aerial spraying of agricultural crops (65). In most industrialized countries the concentration of DDT in human milk has significantly decreased since the enforcement of severe restrictions in its use. In most developing countries, where DDT has been widely used both as an agricultural insecticide and in malaria-control programmes, it is now used much less frequently because of the resistance that insects have developed. In highly contaminated areas DDT is also found in cow's milk. However, industrially prepared breast-milk substitutes are low in, or entirely free of, DDT to the extent that the fat used is uncontaminated and pollution of the products from other sources is controlled.

Although DDT has a relatively low level of toxicity for human adults, it can cause such severe and undesirable effects in animals as hepatic dysfunction and carcinogenesis, and, in birds, disruption of the reproductive rate by causing eggshell thinning and embryo deaths (66). In contrast, the main known effect in mammals, for example bats, is to increase the mortality of migrating adults (66). No information is available concerning the possible deleterious consequences for infants of these levels of DDT. No ill effects associated with breast-feeding have been observed, even in areas of high contamination, but this does not preclude the possibility of long-term consequences.

Maximum daily intakes of DDT and related compounds have been fixed by WHO and other agencies (67, 68). These limits have been set much lower than those of known toxicity. This explains why infants who may be ingesting larger amounts of DDT may still appear to be unharmed.

In cases where there is a high degree of pollution from chemical sources occurring simultaneously in a bacterially contaminated environment, the choice is not simply between polluted breast milk and "risk-free" substitutes (69, 70). Rather, informed choice is based on assessing the known and unknown risks of artificial feeding versus the unknown, but potential, risks of chemical contamination of breast milk. Clearly, the possible toxicity of DDT and similar compounds requires further investigation. Of much greater importance, however, are effective measures to protect the environment for the entire population by controlling the use of these toxic products.

While a marked reduction in the presence and concentration of DDT in human milk has been observed in industrialized countries, other industrial chemicals of a similar nature are causing concern as environmental pollutants. For example, polychlorinated biphenyls (PCBs), which are toxic, non-biologically degradable and fat-soluble chemicals, have been widely used in the manufacture of electrical equipment and hydraulic machines. Environmental contamination from PCBs is common the world over, and they accumulate in the body and are excreted only in milk (71). Although their industrial use is now restricted, environmental contamination will persist for some time, since there are no practical, economical means for eliminating these very stable chemicals.

Products of even higher toxicity such as polychlorinated dioxins (PCDDs) and furans (PCDFs) (72) can be produced accidentally through fires and explosions in electrical equipment. It has also been determined that most incinerators produce these environmental contaminants.

There is no scientific evidence of any undesirable effects in infants resulting from the ingestion of these pollutants via breast milk, in which they are found usually in low concentrations. However, not enough experience has been gained to exclude the possibility of long-term effects, particularly to exposure through prolonged breast-feeding. Overall, the advantages of breast-feeding are still considered to be greater than the potential risks, particularly during the first months of life.

In a number of industrialized countries, where it is assumed that breast-feeding after four months is less critical to infant health than in some societies, there has been some discussion of the possibility of counselling mothers against prolonged lactation to avoid an accumulation of fat-soluble contaminants in their infants. On the basis of present scientific knowledge, however, such a measure does not appear justified. In fact, the concentration of fat-soluble contaminants in breast milk decreases as lactation advances, and with increasing parity (72, 73).

Smoking increases the exposure of mothers and infants to many chemical compounds, including pesticide residues and known carcinogens. It is associated with higher levels of chemical contaminants in milk as well as reduced duration of breast-feeding (74) and higher levels of infant distress ("colic") (75). Because of its well-known adverse health consequences for both mothers and infants (76), women who smoke should be encouraged to breast-feed and to eliminate, or at least reduce, cigarette use during pregnancy and lactation.

Another pregnancy. Although there are many taboos and cultural beliefs against breast-feeding when the woman concerned becomes pregnant again, breast-feeding during pregnancy is still a fairly common practice in many societies. Supposed changes in breast-milk volume or composition associated with a new pregnancy have not been confirmed by factual observations. No ill effects have been detected either for the mother or the infant, although many mothers wean voluntarily either because their children lose interest or the mothers develop painful nipples. The main concern in such situations is whether the mother's additional nutritional requirements are being met (see chapters 1 and 2).

It is highly unlikely that a lactating woman will become pregnant before her child has begun to be weaned. Usually, it is only when the child is receiving significant amounts of complementary foods, and therefore the frequency and intensity of sucking has decreased, that she becomes pregnant again. In traditional societies this rarely occurs before the infant reaches the age of six months. Another three months will usually elapse before the mother realizes that she is pregnant, and only then does she face the decision of continuing to breast-feed or not. By this time the infant has benefited from the period when breast-feeding is of greatest value and family foods can be more easily and safely introduced.

Problems in this context arise among populations that consume mainly staple foods that are nutritionally inadequate or otherwise inappropriate for infant feeding, e.g., cassava, plantain and maize, with practically no products of animal origin. Under such conditions, however, the problem is more one of identifying appropriate weaning foods than of replacing breast milk. Supplementing the mother's own diet with commonly available foods is certainly preferable to interrupting lactation on account of a new pregnancy, particularly when an adequate weaning diet cannot be ensured.

Malnutrition. In extremely undernourished mothers, for example during famine conditions, breast-milk secretion decreases and may stop completely. From a practical point of view, however, it is more important to understand whether, and at what point, milk volume and composition are affected in mothers who are in a chronic state of mild-to-moderate malnutrition.

It is believed that a large proportion of women in some developing countries, although not presenting clear clinical signs of malnutrition, are to varying degrees nutrient- or energy-deficient. The effects of this situation on lactation performance are extremely difficult to assess, let alone quantify, for lack of adequate methods for diagnosing mild-to-moderate subclinical forms of malnutrition. Moreover, malnutrition does not occur in isolation, but is usually observed simultaneously with other variables that may themselves influence lactation performance. Some of these variables will have a positive bearing, for example the fact that breast-feeding is the traditional way of feeding infants and is, therefore, protected and supported by society as a whole. Others, such as hard physical labour and environmental stress, may exercise a negative influence.

Both types of variables tend to invalidate comparisons between populations living under very different socioeconomic and environmental conditions. There are reports of infants in conditions of poverty whose growth falters earlier than would be expected for the fully breast-fed (77), and of seasonal variations in milk output associated with changes in the dietary intake of mothers (78). Nevertheless, the fact remains that the vast majority of mothers who live in socially and economically deprived circumstances, and who are considered to be suffering from varying degrees of chronic malnutrition, are able to breast-feed their infants successfully and for long periods.

The difficulties associated with assessing maternal nutritional status (see chapter 1), together with the possible influence of other variables, may account for the inconclusive results of studies of the effect on lactation performance of the supplementary feeding of mothers. Maternal nutrition during pregnancy helps to determine lactation performance. Thus, food supplementation during lactation may not produce the desired results if a mother's dietary intake was deficient during pregnancy.

In the WHO study concerning the quantity and quality of breast milk in different countries and at various socioeconomic levels (79), it was found that only among poor rural women in Zaire were there any indications of reduced milk production possibly associated with poor maternal nutritional status. Nevertheless, these same mothers were able to secrete consistently the same amount of breast milk throughout the first eighteen months of their children's lives. Poor rural women in Guatemala and the Philippines produced no less milk than their well-to-do urban counterparts, and, as with women in Zaire, they maintained milk production well beyond the first year of their children's lives. The introduction of other foods into the infant diet appears to be the main factor associated with decreased breast-milk secretion. For example, lactation performance was poor from the first month among the well-to-do urban mothers surveyed in the Philippines, who were also the most frequent users of breast-milk substitutes (79).

As to composition, available evidence suggests that maternal diet and nutritional status have very little influence on the macronutrient content (carbohydrates, proteins and fats)—and therefore energy concentration—of breast milk (79). It appears that, whereas the quantity of milk may decrease if there are not enough "raw materials" available to the mammary gland, its composition at least is not significantly altered.

The situation is different where micronutrients (vitamins and minerals) are concerned, their presence in breast milk being directly influenced by a mother's own nutritional status. The development of beriberi in infants of thiamine-deficient mothers is a typical example of this relationship. In the WHO study (79), no significant differences were found between various groups as regards the energy content and the main constituents of breast milk. The single exception to this rule—a higher energy content of the milk—among well-to-do urban mothers, compared with poor rural mothers, was identified in Sweden but not in Guatemala and the Philippines.

In conclusion, nutritional deficiencies that are believed to be widespread among the world's women merit continued close attention, for the improvement of their own health and that of their infants. As a general rule, however, mild-to-moderate subclinical forms of malnutrition are not an indication for these mothers not to breast-feed their infants. In fact, not breast-feeding under such circumstances may only worsen the situation for the infant in question, who is deprived of breast milk's many benefits, as well as for the other family members when scarce resources are used to provide a nutritionally adequate substitute.

Perceived milk insufficiency. As mentioned earlier, only in exceptional circumstances, for example inborn errors of metabolism, will a mother's milk be inadequate for the healthy growth and development of her infant. Many mothers nevertheless decide to complement the diets of their breast-fed infants, or to stop breast-feeding altogether, either because they believe that they are not producing enough milk or that their milk is inadequate to meet their infants' nutritional needs. Mothers who consider that their milk is "too thin", for example, may be comparing it to cow's milk, which is quite different in appearance.

As with lactation failure (also discussed above), perceived milk insufficiency occurs most frequently among educated, healthy and well-nourished mothers for whom there is virtually no physiological evidence of low milk productivity, and still less for inadequate milk composition. The real stumbling block is frequently related to emotional and psychosocial factors, or to an incomplete understanding of the mechanics of lactation and breast-feeding techniques. An infant's health status and weight gain should provide such mothers with convincing evidence of the sufficient quantity and nutritional adequacy of their breast milk.

The problem of perceived milk insufficiency, however, may be no less real in its consequences as a result of stress, which can interfere with the "let-down" reflex (see chapter 2). Inadequate sucking by the infant due to inappropriate feeding techniques (e.g., improper positioning (*80*)) and subsidiary difficulties related to breast-feeding that go unresolved for lack of proper guidance and support can also lead to insufficient milk. Often, the very complementary foods that were introduced because of unfounded fears about the quality and quantity of breast milk contribute directly to decreased milk secretion.

Résumé

Les facteurs pouvant interférer avec l'allaitement maternel

Un régime équilibré est essentiel durant la petite enfance, toute anomalie nutritionnelle étant davantage ressentie par le nourrisson, beaucoup moins adaptable qu'un sujet plus âgé. L'allaitement maternel est le meilleur moyen d'assurer la croissance et le développement sains des enfants normaux. Il y a cependant un certain nombre de situations, heureusement rares, où les nourrissons ne peuvent ou ne doivent être nourris au sein. Ce chapitre examine les situations où l'allaitement maternel est contre-indiqué pour des raisons liées soit à la santé de l'enfant soit à celle de la mère et où par conséquent des substituts du lait maternel peuvent être indiqués pendant de longues périodes. Il faut aussi distinguer entre les enfants qui ne doivent pas du tout recevoir de lait maternel et ceux qui ne peuvent être nourris au sein mais pour lesquels le lait maternel est néanmoins l'aliment de choix. Il y a aussi ceux qui ne tolèrent aucun lait et qui ont besoin de préparations nutritives spéciales. Le cas des enfants de faible poids de naissance est envisagé au chapitre 5.

Raisons liées à la santé de l'enfant

Erreurs innées du métabolisme. Certaines maladies métaboliques héréditaires ou congénitales associées à une anomalie enzymatique spécifique rendent impossible la consommation de certains éléments du lait. Trois de ces maladies sont particulièrement importantes: la galactosémie, la phénylcétonurie et la maladie du sirop d'érable. Des malformations congénitales comme le bec de lièvre et les fentes palatines peuvent aussi être à l'origine de problèmes de succion.

Raisons liées à la santé de la mère

Carence de la lactation. Elle doit être distinguée du sentiment souvent décrit par les mères de manquer de lait. Elle se rencontre généralement dans les pays industrialisés, chez des mères par ailleurs en bonne santé sans raisons physiologiques apparentes expliquant l'absence de sécrétion lactée. Les facteurs psychosociaux semblent jouer un grand rôle mais sont difficiles à identifier.

Maladies de la mère

L'allaitement au sein est contre-indiqué dans le cas d'affections graves du coeur (insuffisance cardiaque) du foie, du rein ou du poumon ou dans le cas de malnutrition sévère, par exemple lors d'une famine. Le problème de la transmission de maladies infectieuses reste cependant préoccupant et ce chapitre donne des détails sur certains aspects:

— les mastites en particulier à *Staphylococcus aureus* ne doivent pas faire interrompre l'allaitement. Les abcès du sein qui sont souvent des complications de ces mastites apparaissent aussi après un arrêt brutal de l'allaitement au sein mais ne sont pas non plus des causes d'interruption;
— une tuberculose évolutive qui doit être diagnostiquée et traitée;
— parmi les infections virales le chapitre met l'accent entre autres sur les infections à cytomégalovirus qui ne doivent pas empêcher l'allaitement, l'herpès simple qui demande des précautions d'hygiène accrues mais non l'arrêt du lait maternel, l'hépatite B où la transmission de la mère infectée à son nouveau-né par le lait ne peut être exclue mais où l'allaitement maternel doit être poursuivi, assorti de certaines précautions comme aux USA, où la prévalence des porteurs est pourtant inférieure à 1%;
— le virus HIV. Le virus HIV a été cultivé à partir du lait de mères infectées. Il semble que le risque additionnel apporté par l'allaitement maternel soit minime et limité à certaines circonstances particulières. Parmi les femmes infectées mais asymptomatiques, compte non tenu du risque d'une transmission intra-utérine, l'allaitement maternel ne paraît pas augmenter le risque d'une infection de l'enfant. Le lait maternel peut être aussi important dans la prévention d'infections intercurrentes qui pourraient accélérer l'évolution d'affections opportunistes chez les nourrissons déjà infectés.

Les recommandations formulées lors d'une

réunion technique organisée par l'OMS en 1987 demeurent valables, à savoir: l'allaitement maternel doit continuer de recevoir la protection, l'encouragement et le soutien qu'il mérite à cause de tous les bénéfices qu'il apporte (voir chapitre 2) et ceci aussi bien dans les pays en développement que dans ceux qui sont industrialisés. Dans de nombreuses circonstances, en particulier quand il n'existe pas d'autres solutions à la fois efficaces et sûres, l'allaitement fourni par la mère biologique doit être la méthode de choix, quel que soit l'état d'infection vis à vis du virus HIV.

Facteurs qui ne sont pas normalement considérés comme contraires à l'allaitement maternel

Facteurs liés à l'enfant. Grossesses multiples, ictère du lait de femme, hémorragies du nouveau-né, diarrhée.

Facteurs liés à la mère. Cancer du sein, inversion du mamelon, thérapie médicamenteuse (la prise de médicaments devrait être évitée chez les mères allaitantes);

— pollution chimique de l'environnement. On retrouve dans le lait de nombreux composés chimiques, en particulier des résidus d'insecticides chlorés comme le DDT qui sont hautement toxiques. Ces produits sont excrétés dans le lait, concentrés dans les graisses. Il n'existe pas d'information sur les effets toxiques du DDT trouvé dans le lait maternel. On n'a pas signalé d'effets pathologiques mais rien n'indique qu'il ne puisse y avoir d'effets à long terme;
— autre grossesse;
— malnutrition.

Une production de lait insuffisante est souvent alléguée par les mères pour introduire un complément dans l'alimentation de leurs nourrissons. A côté des facteurs affectifs et psychologiques évoqués plus haut, il est de fait que l'anxiété peut altérer le réflexe d'éjection.

References

1. **Lawrence, R.A.** *Breast-feeding: a guide for the medical profession.* St Louis, C.V. Mosby, 1989, p. 347.
2. **Udall, J.N. et al.** Liver disease in alpha 1-antitrypsin deficiency: a retrospective analysis of the influence of early breast- versus bottle-feeding. *J. Am. Med. Assoc.,* **253**: 2679–2692 (1985).
3. **Edelstein, D. et al.** The removal of lactose from human milk by fermentation with *Saccharomyces fragilis. Milchwissenschaft,* **34**: 733 (1979).
4. **Stanbury, J.B. et al.,** ed. *The metabolic basis of inherited disease,* 5th ed. New York, McGraw-Hill, 1983, p. 180.
5. **Berger, L.R.** When should one discourage breast-feeding? *Pediatrics,* **67**: 300–302 (1981).
6. **Francis, D.E.M.** *Diets for sick children.* Oxford, Blackwell Scientific Publications, 1987.
7. **Stanbury, J.B. et al.,** see ref. *4,* p. 279.
8. **Tsang, R.C. & Nichols, B.L.,** ed. *Nutrition during infancy.* St Louis, C.V. Mosby, 1988.
9. **Naylor, E.W. & Guthrie, R.** Newborn screening for maple-syrup urine disease (branched-chain ketoaciduria). *Pediatrics,* **61**: 262–266 (1978).
10. **Weatherley-White, R.C.A. et al.** Early repair and breast-feeding for infants with cleft lip. *Plastic and reconstr. surg.,* **79**: 879–885 (1987).
11. **Behrman, R.E. & Vaughan, V.C.,** ed. *Nelson's Textbook of Pediatrics.* Philadelphia, W.B. Saunders, 1983, p. 881.
12. *Contemporary patterns of breast-feeding.* Geneva, World Health Organization, 1981.
13. **Mata, L.J.** *The children of Santa Maria Cauque.* Cambridge, MA, MIT Press, 1978, p. 202.
14. **Houston, M.J. & Field, P.A.** Practices and policies in the initiation of breast-feeding. *J. obstet. gynecol. neonat. nut.,* **17**: 418–424 (1988).
15. **Garforth, S. & Garcia, J.** Breast-feeding policies in practice—"No wonder they get confused!" *Midwifery,* **5**: 75–83 (1989).
16. **Neifert, M.R.** Infant problems in breast-feeding. In: Neville, M.C. & Neifert, M.R., ed. *Lactation.* New York, Plenum Press, 1983.
17. **Lawrence, R.A.,** see ref. *1,* pp. 156–158 & 409–410.
18. **Chalmers, I. et al.** *Effective care in pregnancy and childbirth.* Oxford, Oxford University Press, 1989.
19. **Minchin, M.K.** *Breastfeeding matters.* Melbourne, Alma Publications, 1989, ch. 6.
20. **Porter, P.** Adoptive immunization of the neonate by breast factors. In: Ogra, P.L. & Dayton, D.H., ed. *Immunology of breast milk.* New York, Raven Press, 1979.
21. **Thomsen, A.C. et al.** Leukocyte counts and microbiological cultivation in the diagnosis of puerperal mastitis. *Am. j. obstet. gynecol.,* **146**: 938–941 (1983).
22. **Thomsen, A.C. et al.** Course and treatment of milk stasis, noninfectious inflammation of the breast, and infectious mastitis in nursing women. *Am. j. obstet. gynecol.,* **149**: 492–495 (1984).
23. *Tuberculosis control as an integral part of primary health care.* Geneva, World Health Organization, 1988.
24. Prophylaxis with isoniazid. *The Medical Letter,* **30** (No. 763): 44 (1988).
25. **Minchin, M.K.,** see ref. *19,* p. 328.
26. **Reynolds, D.W. et al.** Maternal cytomegalovirus excretion and perinatal infection. *New Engl. j. med.,* **289**: 1–5 (1973).
27. **Pearay, L.O. et al.** Immunology of breast milk: mater-

nal neonatal interactions. In: Freier, S. & Eidelman, A.I., ed. *Human milk. Its biological and social value.* Amsterdam, Excerpta Medica, 1980.

28. **Stagno, S. et al.** Breast milk and the risk of CMV infection. *New Engl. j. med.*, **302**: 1073–1076 (1980).

29. **Dworsky, M. et al.** Cytomegalovirus infection of breast milk and transmission in infancy. *Pediatrics*, **72**: 295–299 (1983).

30. **Boehn, F.H. et al.** Management of genital herpes simplex infection occurring during pregnancy. *Am. j. obst. gynecol*, **141**: 735–740 (1981).

31. **Lee, A.K. et al.** Mechanisms of maternal–fetal transmission of hepatitis B virus. *J. infect. dis.*, **138**. 668–671 (1978).

32. **Stevens, C.E.** Viral hepatitis in pregnancy: the obstetrician's role. *Clin. obstet. gynecol.*, **25**: 577–584 (1982).

33. **American Academy of Pediatrics.** *Report of the Committee on Infectious Diseases*, 19th ed. Edmonton, Illinois, 1982.

34. **Vajro, P. et al.** Breast-feeding enhances the clearance of HBsAg in infants with hepatitis B infection. *Gastroenterology*, **88**: 1702 (abstract) (1985).

35. **Thiry L. et al.** Isolation of AIDS virus from cell-free breast milk of three healthy women carriers. *Lancet*, **2**: 891–892 (1985).

36. **Ziegler, J.B. et al.** Postnatal transmission of AIDS-associated retrovirus from mother to infant. *Lancet*, **1**: 896–897 (1985).

37. **Oxtaby, M.J.** Human immunodeficiency virus and other viruses in human milk: placing the issues in broader perspective. *Pediatr. dis. j.*, **7**: 825–835 (1988).

38. Breast-feeding/breast milk and human immunodeficiency virus (HIV). *Wkly epidem. rec.*, **62**(33): 245–246 (1987).

39. **Global Programme on AIDS.** *Report of the meeting on Criteria for HIV Screening Programmes.* Document WHO/SPA/GLO/87.2. Geneva, World Health Organization, 1987.

40. **Hartmann, P.E. & Kent, J.C.** The subtlety of breast milk. *Breast-feeding review*, **13**: 14–18 (1988).

41. **Prentice, A. et al.** Dietary supplementation of lactating Gambian women. Effect on breast-milk volume and quality. *Human nut.: clin. nutr.*, **37**(C): 53–64 (1983).

42. **Prentice, A. et al.** Cross-cultural differences in lactational performance. In: Hamosh, M. & Goldman, A.S., ed. *Human lactation, 2: maternal and environmental factors.* New York, Plenum Press, 1986.

43. **Hopkinson, J.M. et al.** Milk production by mothers of premature infants. *Pediatrics*, **81**: 815–820 (1988).

44. **Auerbach, K.G. & Gartner, L.M.** Breast-feeding and human milk: their association with jaundice in the neonate. *Clin. perinatol.*, **14**: 89–108 (1987).

45. **Gartner, L.M. & Lee, K.S.** Jaundice and liver disease. In: Behrman, R.E. et al., ed. *Neonatal-perinatal medical diseases of the fetus and infant*, 2nd ed. St Louis, C.V. Mosby, 1977.

46. **Stocker, R. et al.** Bilirubin is an anti-oxidant of possible physiological importance. *Science*, **235**: 1043–1046 (1987).

47. **Gartner, L.M. & Arias, I.M.** Temporary discontinuation of breast-feeding in infants with jaundice. *J. Am. Med. Assoc.*, **225**: 532–533 (1973).

48. **Gleason, W.A. & Kerr, G.R.** Questions about quinones in infant nutrition. *J. pediatr. gastroenterol. nutr.*, **8**: 285–287 (1989).

49. **Greer, F.R. & Suttle, J.W.** Vitamin K and the newborn. In: Tsang, R.C. & Nichols, B.L., ed., see ref. *8*, p. 295.

50. **U, K.M. et al.** Effect on clinical outcome of breast-feeding during acute diarrhoea. *Br. med. j.*, **290**: 587–589 (1985).

51. **Byers, T. et al.** Lactation and breast cancer: evidence for a negative association in premenopausal women. *Am. j. epidemiol.*, **121**: 664–674 (1985).

52. **McTiernan, A. & Thomas, D.B.** Evidence for a protective effect of lactation on risk of breast cancer in young women: results from a case-control study. *Am. j. epidemiol*, **124**. 353–358 (1986).

53. **Kvale, G. & Heuch, I.J.** Lactation and cancer risk: is there a relation specific to breast cancer? *J. epidemiol. comm. health*, **42**: 30–37 (1988).

54. **Fraumeni, J.F. & Miller, R.W.** Breast cancer from breast-feeding. *Lancet*, **2**: 1196–1197 (1971).

55. **Lawrence, R.A.**, see ref. *1*, pp. 183–186.

56. **Hoffman, J.B.** A suggested treatment for inverted nipples. *Am. j. obst. gynecol.*, **66**: 346–348 (1953).

57. **Waller, H.** The early failure of breast-feeding. *Arch. dis. childhood*, **21**: 1–12 (1946).

58. **Wilson, J.T.**, ed. *Drugs in breast milk.* Lancaster, MTP Press, 1981.

59. **Briggs, G.G. et al.** *Drugs in pregnancy and lactation.* Amsterdam, Elsevier, 1988.

60. **Bennett, P.N. et al.** *Drugs and human lactation.* Amsterdam, Elsevier, 1988.

61. **American Academy of Pediatrics: Committee on Drugs.** The transfer of drugs and other chemicals into human breast milk. *Pediatrics*, **72**: 375–383 (1983).

62. Breast-feeding and fertility regulation: current knowledge and programme policy implications. *Bull. Wld Hlth Org.*, **61**: 371–382 (1983).

63. **Betrabet, S.S. et al.** Transfer of norethisterone (NET) and levonorgestrel (LNG) from a single tablet into the infant's circulation through the mother's milk. *Contraception*, **35**: 517–522 (1987).

64. Consensus Statement. Breast-feeding as a family planning method. *Lancet*, **2**: 1204–1205 (1988).

65. **Olzyna-Marzys, A.E.** Contaminants in human milk. *Acta paediatrica Scandinavica*, **67**: 571–576 (1978).

66. *DDT and its derivatives—environmental aspects.* (Environmental Health Criteria 83). Geneva, World Health Organization, 1989, p. 11.

67. **Food and Agriculture Organization, World Health Organization.** *Evaluation of some pesticide residues in food.* FAO/AGP/1970/M 12/1; WHO/Food Add./71.42 (1970).

68. **Food and Drug Administration.** *Food and Drug Administration action levels for poisonous or deleterious substances in human food and animal feed.* Washington, DC, 1978.

69. **Muytjens, H.L. et al.** Quality of powdered substitutes for breast milk with regard to members of the family

Enterobacteriaceae. J. clin. microbiol., **26**: 743–746 (1988).

70. **Minchin, M.K.** Infant formula: a mass uncontrolled trial in perinatal care. *Birth*, **14**: 97–105 (1987).

71. *Assessment of health risks in infants associated with exposure to PCBs, PCDDs and PCDFs in breast milk.* (Environmental Health Series 29). Copenhagen, World Health Organization, 1988.

72. **Stacey, I.S. & Tatum, T.** House treatment with organochlorine pesticides and their levels in human milk in Perth, Western Australia. *Bull. environ. toxicol.*, **35**: 202–208 (1985).

73. **Rogan, W.J. et al.** Polychlorinated biphenyls (PCBs) and dichlorodiphenyl dichloroethane (DDE) in human milk: effects of maternal factors and previous lactation. *Am. j. pub. health*, **76**: 172–177 (1986).

74. **Woodward, A. & Hand, K.** Smoking and reduced duration of breast-feeding. *Med. j. Austr.*, **148**: 477–478 (1988).

75. **Said, G. et al.** Infantile colic and parental smoking. *Br. med. j.*, **289**: 660 (1984).

76. Population Reports, Series L, No. 1. *Tobacco—hazards to health and human reproduction.* Baltimore, Johns Hopkins University, 1979.

77. **Habicht, J.-P. et al.** Height and weight standards for preschool children. How relevant are ethnic differences in growth potential? *Lancet*, **1**: 611–615 (1974).

78. **Paul, A.A. et al.** The quantitative effects of maternal dietary intake on pregnancy and lactation in rural Gambian women. *Trans. Roy. Soc. Trop. Med. Hyg.*, **73**: 686–692 (1979).

79. *The quantity and quality of breast milk. Report on the WHO Collaborative Study on Breast-feeding.* Geneva, World Health Organization, 1985.

80. **Minchin, M.K.** Position for breastfeeding: commentary and reply. *Birth*, **16**: 67–80 (1989).

4. Physiological development of the infant and its implications for complementary feeding

From the standpoint of nutritional needs, physiological maturation, and immunological safety the provision of foods other than breast milk before about four months of age is unnecessary and may also be harmful. On the other hand, many infants require some complementary feeding by about six months of age. There are a number of known disadvantages and risks involved in too early complementary feeding, including interference with the infant's feeding behaviour, reduced breast-milk production, decreased iron absorption from breast milk, increased risk of infections and allergy in infants, and increased risk of a new pregnancy. With many complementary foods, including undiluted cow's milk, there is also a risk of a water deficit with a resultant hyperosmolarity and hypernatraemia that, in extreme cases, can lead to lethargy, convulsions, and even residual brain damage. Other possible implications include the development of obesity, hypertension, and arteriosclerosis in later life. The decision about when to start complementary feeding depends not only on age but also on the developmental stage of the individual infant, the type of food available, the sanitary conditions in which the food is prepared and given, and family history of atopic disease.

Introduction

During the intrauterine period, the fetus is "fed" through the placental circulation. As briefly discussed in chapter 1, the placenta transmits from the mother's blood all required nutrients, which directly enter the fetal circulation in an immediately usable form. Glucose is the main source of energy, while free amino acids are used for protein synthesis. Owing to this mechanism the fetus does not have to ingest, digest and absorb food, nor is an excretory system required. Whatever waste is produced goes back into the mother's circulation. The gastrointestinal tract and renal functions develop progressively prior to birth, in preparation for the day when they will be needed.

There is evidence that, late in pregnancy, the fetus demonstrates swallowing movements and takes in amniotic fluid; this has very little, if any, nutritional significance, though it is of importance for the anatomical and functional development of the fetal gastrointestinal system. Similarly, the fetus produces and excretes urine, which passes into the amniotic fluid even though the kidneys are still developing and are not yet playing a vital role.

The situation changes radically at birth, after which the infant must take food by mouth, digest and absorb the nutrients, and have functioning kidneys to excrete metabolic wastes and maintain water and electrolyte homeostasis. However, since neither the digestive nor excretory system is as yet fully developed, the margin of tolerance for water, overall solute load, and specific solutes is very narrow compared with the older infant and young child. Because of the inability of the kidneys to concentrate urine at birth and for several months thereafter, the neonate

and young infant require food with a higher water content than that taken by the older infant in order to be able to excrete a comparable solute load.

The process of adaptation to these drastic changes occurs during the first few months of extrauterine life, during which the infant is also growing rapidly and therefore has high nutritional requirements. Both the sucking and extrusion reflexes, present at birth and active throughout the first months of life, prime the infant to receive only liquid nourishment. If other foods are given at this time, they are usually regurgitated.

Appropriate feeding practices during the first months of life are thus conditioned by the infant's nutritional needs and degree of functional maturity, particularly as regards the types of food, mechanism of excretion and defences against infection. This chapter reviews the development of the gastrointestinal tract and renal functions during early extrauterine life and the corresponding nutritional needs. It also considers infant-feeding practices, particularly complementary feeding.

Gastrointestinal-tract functions

Food ingestion

At birth the normal infant is able to suck from the mother's breast, conduct the milk thus obtained to the back of the mouth and swallow it. The infant can do this for five to ten minutes continuously while breathing normally. As discussed in chapter 2, the sucking and swallowing functions are vital for the newborn and the infant during the first months of life. They are achieved by a special morphological configuration of the mouth, with, in particular, a proportionately longer soft palate than is found later in life, and by the sucking and swallowing reflexes, which direct a series of coordinated movements of the lips, cheeks, tongue and pharynx. By six months of age, the ability to swallow fluids offered by cup has begun to develop.

If solid or semi-solid food is placed in the young infant's mouth, it is normally vigorously rejected by the action of another of the infant's normal reflexes. It is only at four to six months of age, when the tongue thrust, or extrusion reflex, is normally no longer present, that the infant is able to cope with semi-solid foods; hence the food can be transported to the rear of the mouth and swallowed (1). The series of movements needed for this purpose are different from those needed for sucking and swallowing liquids. Later, at seven to nine months of age, rhythmic biting movements start to appear at the same time as the first teeth are erupting; mastication has begun.

For the first four to six months of life the normal infant is thus at a stage of functional development that allows the acceptance of an essentially liquid diet. This is a period of transition between the fetal nutrition *in utero* and the mixed, mainly solid, diet of later life. While a young infant can be forced to take soft semi-solid foods from the first days after birth, for example by a mother who learns how to utilize the infant's sucking movements to feed such foods, this cannot be considered either normal or desirable.

Food digestion

Carbohydrates. The process of food digestion starts in the mouth; during mastication foods are mixed with saliva allowing the action of amylase to begin the digestion of starches. Although amylase has been found in infant saliva, no digestion of carbohydrates takes place in the mouth or oesophagus during the first months of life.

Carbohydrates are digested mainly in the proximal small intestine. Polysaccharides, like starches, are degraded into mono- and disaccharides, primarily by the action of delta-amylase secreted by the pancreas. Glucoamylase secreted by the intestinal mucosa may also contribute to the digestion of starches, but it acts primarily on oligosaccharides and some disaccharides. The small intestine's mucosa also secretes disaccharidases, which hydrolyse disaccharides into monosaccharides, the only form in which carbohydrates can be absorbed.

It has been determined that infants born at term have approximately 10% of adult amylase activity in their small intestine (2) and this seems to be mainly glucoamylase activity. Present information indicates that pancreatic amylase is not secreted during the first three months of life; it has been found to be present only at very low levels, or absent altogether, up to six months of age (3).

There is, however, some evidence that infants can digest starches before three months of age. This is probably due to the activity of glucoamylase, which is not normally active at this time, but which is activated by the presence and nature of the substance or substrate on which the enzyme acts (4). It is also possible that pancreatic amylase could be produced as a reaction to the presence of starches in the small intestine, although this has not been proved. In any case, a process of adaptation is required for the young infant to be able to digest starches. This can take days or weeks and might explain the frequency with which gastrointestinal disturbances, particularly diarrhoea, are observed in small infants fed starch-containing foods. It has also been suggested that undigested starches may interfere with the absorption of other nutrients and result in failure to thrive in infants fed diets containing a large proportion of starches (5).

Contrary to the evident immaturity of the infant's system for the digestion and utilization of starches during the first months of life, the activity of the disaccharidases is fully developed at birth. Both delta-glucosidase, which hydrolyses sucrose and maltose, and beta-galactosidase, which hydrolyses lactose, are present at birth at the same activity levels as those found in older infants (6). The digestion and utilization of milk sugar, therefore, poses no problem at this age.

Proteins. The gastric secretion of hydrochloric acid and pepsin is already well developed in the newborn at term; concentrations are low, however, and increase progressively during the first months of life (7, 8). In any case, the digestion of proteins takes place mainly in the small intestine, where proteolytic activity in the newborn has reached the same concentration as in adults (9). Thus, while the young infant may have some difficulty with proteins like casein for which gastric activity can be important to initiate digestion, the infant's capacity to digest proteins is otherwise fully developed at birth. Nevertheless, very high protein intake should be avoided, particularly in the pre-term and very young infant, in whom an excessive renal solute load may produce acid-base imbalances and metabolic acidosis.

Another problem related to the young infant's use of proteins is the permeability of the intestinal mucosa to large molecules. In older infants, as in adults, proteins are absorbed as amino acids and small peptides. Most of the latter are further digested during their passage through the mucosa, and it is mainly the free amino acids which enter the circulation. Large molecules, which can act as antigens, do not normally cross the intestinal mucosa. During the neonatal period, however, and for a variable time thereafter, the infant is able to absorb protein molecules intact (10), as demonstrated by the absorption of antibodies and the immunological response to protein antigens administered orally.

This physiological characteristic of the young infant seems to be one mechanism by which an allergic reaction to cow's milk sometimes develops in children. Its implications for the development of other food allergies is not clear but should be borne in mind when decisions about the feeding of young infants are being made.

Fats. As mentioned above, glucose is the main source of energy for fetal development during the intra-uterine period. After birth, however, dietary fats become an important energy source. Some 40–50% of energy in human milk is in the form of fats. A drastic adjustment in energy metabolism is therefore required after birth, starting with the digestion and absorption of fats.

In older infants and adults, dietary fats are first hydrolysed, mainly by the activity of the pancreatic lipases in the small intestine. The products of lipolysis are then solubilized for absorption by the action of the bile salts. In the newborn at term, the pancreatic and hepatic functions are not yet fully developed and the concentrations of both pancreatic lipase and bile salts are very low (11, 12).

It has been observed, however, that young infants adequately absorb fats, particularly those from human milk. This is somewhat surprising considering that milk-fat droplets are particularly resistant to the lipolytic activity of pancreatic lipases because they are enveloped by a layer of phospholipids and proteins. It is known that fat digestion and absorption in young infants are enhanced by the action of lingual lipases (13) and by the action of a lipase contained in human milk (14). Lingual lipases are secreted by papillae on the posterior part of the tongue; they start to act in the stomach and the products of lipolysis (fatty acids and monoglycerides) contribute to the emulsification of the mixture, thereby compensating for low bile-salt content. This important mechanism of preduodenal lipolysis in the young infant is further complemented by the lipase contained in breast milk (bile-salt stimulated lipase), which also plays an important role during early infancy in fat digestion and absorption. The breast-milk lipase also has esterase activity, which is vital for utilization of vitamin A that is present in milk in the form of retinol esters.

In spite of the immaturity of the pancreatic and hepatic functions, the young infant is thus well equipped to make use of both the fat in breast milk, which provides close to half of energy requirements, and its other important fat-soluble components. These compensatory, or complementary, mechanisms for fat utilization are less efficient when cow's-milk fat or other fats are introduced into the young infant's diet (15).

Vitamins and minerals. There appear to be no major problems in the utilization of dietary vitamins and minerals in early life. However, the subject has not been studied as much as the digestion and utilization of the macronutrients already discussed. The absorption of fat-soluble vitamins is closely linked to fat absorption. For vitamin A in particular, not enough is known about the utilization by young infants of the different forms in which it or its precursors can occur in foods. The particularly high absorbability of vitamin A in human milk has already been mentioned.

The situation is similar for iron, the absorption of which is higher in infants than in older children and adults. This seems to be related to a greater need for the mineral in early life. In addition, the bio-availability of iron is much higher from breast milk than from cow's milk or preparations added to food (16). The responsible mechanism is not known, although it has been observed that the high bio-availability of breast-milk iron decreases drastically when solid complementary foods of vegetable origin are given to the breast-fed infant. This situation has been confirmed experimentally by measuring, in adults, the iron absorption from breast milk alone or when fed together with a common complementary infant food (strained pears). Iron absorption was found to be 23.8% in the former and 5.7% in the latter case (17).

Water and electrolytes. The permeability of the intestinal mucosa to water and electrolytes is higher during infancy than in later life. This is of no significance under normal conditions but becomes important in situations of high osmolarity in the intestinal contents. Under these circumstances the infant tends to develop water and electrolyte imbalances more easily than later in life, and the implications for infant feeding should thus be carefully borne in mind.

Excretory system

Maintaining the amount and composition of body fluids and excreting metabolic wastes are among the kidneys' vital functions. *In utero* urine formation starts early in fetal development, i.e., by the ninth or

Table 4.1: **Nutrient content of some complementary foods for infants**

A. Macronutrients: average content per 100 g

Product[a]	Country	Industrial (IN) or home-made (HM)	Energy kcal	Energy kJ	Water (%)	Protein (g)	Fat Total (g)	Fat PUFA[b]	Carbohydrates Total (g)	Fibre	Starch
Carrot purée (1)	Sweden	IN	50	200	77.6	1.0	2.0	0.12	7.0	0.77	1.7
Apple purée (2)	England	IN	59	253	—[c]	0.2	ND[d]	ND	15.6	—	—
Rice/milk gruel (powder) (3)	Fed. Rep. of Germany	IN	423	1795	—	10.7	8.9	1.3	75.0	0.1	33.0
Mixed cereals (4)	Netherlands	IN	354	1505	—	10.0	2.0	—	74.0	6.5	—
High protein cereal (5)[e]	USA	IN	360	1512	6.8	35.2	4.6	—	44.3	2.4	—
Chicken/vegetables/potatoes (1)	Sweden	IN	75	320	—	3.0	3.0	—	8.5	—	—
Sweet potatoes (6)	Jamaica	HM	119	477	70.6	1.7	0.4	—	26.3	0.7	—
Green beans (7)	Turkey	HM	32	130	90.1	1.9	0.2	0.07	6.1	1.0	3.8
Papaya (6)	Jamaica	HM	39	160	88.7	0.6	0.1	—	10.0	0.5	0.
Peach (7)	Turkey	HM	38	160	89.1	0.6	0.1	0.05	9.7	0.6	—
Fruit (5)'	USA	IN	85	357	78.2	0.4	0.2	—	20.4	0.5	—
Rice flour/milk/sugar (7)	Turkey	HM	140	586	31.4	2.8	1.2	0.07	28.8	0.07	19.
Corn flour/water (8)	United Rep. of Tanzania	HM	73	304	2.4	1.6	0.5	0.04	15.4	0.14	12.3
Rice/oil/butter/water (9)	India	HM	141	591	3.1	1.9	5.5	1.58	20.3	0.05	20.3
Almond/butter/honey/water (9)	Saudi Arabia	HM	562	2350	11.2	9.5	47.1	6.01	30.4	1.3	9.8
Wheat bread/mint tea (9)	Morocco	HM	288	1210	33.1	8.6	3.8	0.48	53.0	0.2	53.0

B. Minerals: average content per 100 g

Product	Ash (g)	Calcium (mg)	Phosphorus (mg)	Potassium (mg)	Sodium (mg)	Iron (mg)	Copper (mg)	Magnesium (mg)	Zinc (mg)
Carrot purée	0.7	35	30	100	50	0.6	0.06	10	0.20
Apple purée	—	12	5	107	17	0.4	—	—	—
Rice/milk gruel (powder)	—	440	230	430	130	5.0	—	20	—
Mixed cereals	—	50	280	280	260	4.2	—	80	—
High protein cereal[e]	6.7	811	849	1492	68	80.0	0.1	—	0.30
Chicken/vegetables/potatoes	1.0	20	30	170	140	0.7	0.05	10	—
Sweet potatoes	0.7	32	47	243	10	0.7	—	75	—
Green beans	0.6	56	44	243	7	0.8	0.13	32	0.80
Papaya	0.5	20	16	234	3	0.3	0.01	8	0.40
Peach	0.3	9	19	202	1	0.5	—	10	0.5
Fruit'	0.4	8	12	79	17	0.4	0.06	—	—
Rice flour/milk/sugar	0.1	45	53	76	16	0.2	0.01	9	0.50
Corn flour/water	0.2	1	33	ND	ND	0.4	0.03	17	0.28
Rice/oil/butter/water	1.9	15	50	38	53	7.0	0.11	7	0.16
Almod/butter/honey/water	1.5	118	254	403	131	2.5	—	2	1.55
Wheat bread/mint tea		28	94	125	406	5.3	0.13	104	4.39

C. Vitamins: average content per 100 g

	Retinol (eqv. mg)[a]	Vit. D (µg)	Vit. E (mg)	Thiamin (mg)	Riboflavin (mg)	Niacin (mg)	Vit. B$_6$ (mg)	Vit. B$_{12}$ (µg)	Folic acid (µg)	Vit. C (mg)
Carrot purée	1.00	ND	—	0.03	0.03	0.4	—	ND	—	5
Apple purée	—	—	—	—	—	—	—	—	—	25
Rice/milk gruel (powder)	3.30	4.75	3.3	1.3	0.28	2.6	0.24	0.47	47.1	28
Mixed cereals	—	—	—	0.3	0.1	—	0.20	—	—	—
High protein cereal[e]	—	—	—	3.22	1.85	21.0	0.56	—	—	ND
Chicken/vegetables/potatoes	0.10	—	—	0.04	0.02	0.7	—	—	—	21
Sweet potatoes	0.03	ND	—	0.10	0.06	0.6	0.21	ND	88.4	21
Green beans	0.06	ND	0.09	0.08	0.11	0.5	0.15	ND	27.5	19
Papaya	0.18	ND	—	0.04	0.04	0.3	0.04	ND	1.1	56
Peach	0.13	ND	ND	0.02	0.05	1.0	0.02	ND	—	7
Fruit[f]	0.12	—	—	0.02	0.02	0.2	0.05	0.06	0.4	6.8
Rice flour/milk/sugar	0.01	ND	0.07	0.03	0.06	0.4	0.04	ND	1.07	ND
Corn flour/water	ND	ND	ND	0.04	0.01	0.3	0.08	ND	5.3	ND
Rice/oil/butter/water	0.02	ND	0.44	0.11	ND	0.9	0.03	ND	0.9	ND
Almond/butter/honey/water	0.17	0.25	12	0.12	0.48	1.9	0.06	ND	23	ND
Wheat bread/mint tea	ND	ND	1.8	0.27	0.15	3.0	0.26	ND	29	ND

[a] Sources are numbered from 1 to 9 and may be identified from the list given below.

[b] PUFA = polyunsaturated fatty acids.

[c] — = no information available.

[d] ND = none detectable.

[e] Average values of 3 products.

[f] Average values of 33 products.

Sources:

(1) Brown, R.E. Weaning foods in developing countries. *Am. j. clin. nut.*, **31**: 2066–2072 (1978).
(2) Cow & Gate Ltd., Trowbridge, England.
(3) Fomon, S.J. *Infant nutrition*, Philadelphia, Saunders, 1967.
(4) Jelliffe, E.F.P. *A new look at weaning multi-mixes for the Caribbean—means of improving child nutrition*. Jamaica, Caribbean Food and Nutrition Institute, 1971.
(5) Köksal, O. *Nutrition in Turkey*. Ankara, UNICEF, 1977.
(6) Marchione, T.J. & Helsing, E. *Rethinking infant nutrition policies under changing socioeconomic conditions*. University of Oslo, Institute for Nutrition Research, 1981.
(7) International Division/Scientific Department, Milupa, AG, Friedrichsdorf, Federal Republic of Germany.
(8) Nutricia Produktinformatie, Zoetermeer, Netherlands.
(9) Semper Produktinformation, Stockholm, Semper AB, June 1984.

tenth week of gestation. Urine excretion at this stage plays a role in amniotic-fluid maintenance and the embryogenesis of the urinary system. The regulatory and excretory functions of the kidneys are minimal before birth, however, as the task of maintaining fetal homeostasis is carried out by the placenta. Metabolic wastes are practically nil, since fetal metabolism is fundamentally anabolic; whatever waste there is passes through the placenta into the maternal circulation. This is confirmed by the fact that no renal insufficiency is initially evident in infants born with renal agenesis.

At birth the kidneys are performing all their functions but at a limited capacity. They meet the needs of the normal newborn, who continues with a predominantly anabolic metabolism provided that a balanced, fully utilizable, low-residue food, namely breast milk, continues to be fed. The kidneys' functional capability rapidly increases during the first few months of life, as illustrated by their near doubling in size from 12.5 g per kidney at birth to about 20 g at 13 months of age.

The newborn's kidneys are characterized by a low glomerular filtration rate and low concentration capability (18). They function very efficiently, however, as a water-conservation mechanism to prevent dehydration and have no difficulty in eliminating the low metabolic residues of a breast-fed infant. The system can fail when the water intake is markedly reduced or solute intake is noticeably increased. Because the human infant has very different nutritional requirements compared to those of a calf, the giving of undiluted cow's milk can lead to hyperosmolarity with hypernatraemia in the young infant. If not checked, this can result in lethargy, convulsions and even damage to the central nervous system. A cow's-milk diet for the young infant can lead to a water deficit of 80 ml/day. The situation becomes particularly critical when there are extrarenal water losses such as occur with fever or high ambient temperature.

The young infant's kidneys have a limited ability to eliminate hydrogen ions (19), and hence are more susceptible to develop acidosis. Phosphate excretion is a good example of how they adapt their functional capacity to demand. At this age, the kidneys normally function with a low-phosphate intake, as was the case in utero, and should continue this way provided the infant is breast-fed. However, when the infant is put on a high-phosphate diet—cow's milk for instance—the kidneys have to adjust to another level of functioning. Although they usually respond to this demand, it does take time. Meanwhile, the infant may develop transitory hyperphosphataemia as a result of both renal immaturity and functional hypoparathyroidism, which may be associated with hypocalcaemia and neonatal tetany (20).

The relative immaturity of the newborn's renal system seems to be due only to the fact that the level of functioning corresponds to expected demand. The kidneys subsequently mature very rapidly during the first few months of life and are able to adapt to significant variations in diet. Thus, starting at about four months, the solute load resulting from the metabolism of newly introduced foods is acceptable. In fact, progressive modifications in dietary intake, with increments in urea and other solutes to be excreted, stimulate the kidneys to attain higher functional levels. The immature renal system is easily overburdened by such stress situations as disease, dehydration and sudden or too-drastic dietary changes such as the inclusion of foods with high sodium (minerals) or solute loads (proteins), which would require water supplements (see Table 4.1, parts A and B). The use of water with a high mineral content to prepare infant formula is thus undesirable.

Infant feeding

Nutritional requirements

Early life is a period of very rapid growth, with the weight of the normal infant doubling by four months of age. Energy and nutrients are needed not only for maintenance of bodily functions and activity but also, in large proportion, for tissue deposition. Both the quantitative and qualitative nutritional requirements of the infant are consequently different from those of older children and adults. For example, the requirements for both energy and protein during the first month of life are, on a per kilogram basis, about three times those of the adult. There are also other important differences, related either to actual nutritional needs or to the particular physiological characteristics of the infant.

Where proteins are concerned, the requirements of infants for essential amino acids are proportionately much higher than in older children and adults (21, 22). It would therefore by very difficult, if not impossible, to satisfy their nitrogen needs with proteins of low biological value. Fats as such are not required, except for very small amounts of essential fatty acids. Nevertheless, they are extremely important for the infant as a source of concentrated energy, allowing as they do the high-energy intake required within a reasonable volume of food. Mineral requirements are particularly critical at this age; iron and calcium, needed for haemoglobin formation and bone calcification, are notable examples.

More than 50 nutrients are known to be needed by human beings, although information is lacking on the requirements in respect of more than half of them.

For most nutrients there is not only a minimum intake level below which a deficiency occurs but also a maximum level above which they could have undesirable consequences. While the range between these minimum and maximum desirable intakes is quite wide in most cases, it is rather narrow in others. For example, energy-intake levels even slightly below those normally required result in a deficiency while those above will, in time, produce obesity.

A delicate balance of energy and a large number of nutrients is therefore required to ensure appropriate infant nutrition and health. Fortunately, an adequate diet depends less on a consideration of individual nutrients than on the range of foods to be given. For infants up to at least the age of 4–6 months, breast milk is a complete and perfectly balanced mixture of all required nutrients (see chapter 2, on the nutritional quality of breast milk). If the infant's energy needs are satisfied with breast milk, all other nutritional requirements will automatically be met. Exceptions to this rule are infants with very low birth weight who may need iron supplementation (see chapter 5) and infants born of mothers with specific vitamin and mineral deficiencies. In the latter case, a mother's milk may have low values for a given nutrient and her infant may have to be given it as a supplement. The situation is different for infants fed with breast-milk substitutes, who would normally require early supplementation with vitamin C as well as with iron (when the breast-milk substitute used is not enriched with this mineral) and vitamin D (when, because of environmental or other reasons, infants are not exposed to sufficient sunlight) (see Table 4.1, parts B and C).

Energy requirements

Energy requirements can be defined as the level of energy intake from food that will balance the energy expenditure in healthy individuals. Energy expenditure includes the basic metabolism, energy expended in activity, and the energy cost of food utilization. For pregnant and lactating women, the energy cost of pregnancy and lactation has to be added, and for children the energy required for growth.

Ideally, the energy requirement should be determined by accurately measuring all dietary components. While this can usually be done in the case of older children and adults, no reliable information is available on the energy needed by infants for adequate growth and physical activity. However, since it is generally accepted that healthy infants, growing within accepted standards, are in energy balance, the energy intake of such infants has been used as the basis for establishing this group's energy requirements.

Table 4.2: **Energy requirements of infants** (23)

Age (months)	kcal/kg/day	MJ
0–3	120	0.502
3–6	115	0.481
6–9	110	0.460
9–12	105	0.439

To estimate the energy requirements for infants under 6 months of age, an FAO/WHO Ad Hoc Expert Committee on Energy and Protein Requirements (23) in 1971 used data on the intake of infants fed breast milk by bottle and teat (24). For infants 6–12 months of age, data were used concerning healthy children from the USA and the United Kingdom who were fed on a mixed diet (25). Although the information had its limitations, it was the best that was available. The Committee recommended 120 kcal (0.502 MJ) per kg per day for infants 0–3 months of age, decreasing progressively to 105 kcal (0.439 MJ) per kg per day for infants 9–12 months of age (see Table 4.2). It was on this basis that the breast milk of healthy mothers was judged to be insufficient to satisfy the energy requirements of normal infants beyond three months of age (26).

A second consultation, which was jointly sponsored by FAO, WHO and the United Nations University, took place in 1981 to review energy and protein requirements once again (27). This group had access to a much larger collection of food-intake measurements from Canada, Sweden, the United Kingdom and the USA for infants, who were healthy and growing within recommended WHO standards (28). Data from developing countries were intentionally not used in order to exclude any infants growing below the recommended standard, which is associated more with inadequate diet and frequent infections than with genetic differences (29). The interesting results of an analysis of the data used by the 1981 Committee are summarized in Table 4.3.

Although energy intake values start at a level similar to those of the 1971 recommendations, they drop rapidly during the first months of life, beginning to rise again after the tenth month. This U-shaped curve is very different from the progressively decreasing line followed by the 1971 values; it is considered to be more accurate, however, and is probably related to a rapid decline in the energy required for growth. In contrast, energy expenditure through activity, which is initially low, increases progressively to assume greater significance during the latter part of the first year of life. The differences between these observed intake values and the 1971 recommendations are considerable, particularly during the critical period when the weaning process starts. They explain why, under

origins. A better understanding of the etiology and natural history of obesity is important since treatment is difficult once the condition has developed. One of the important questions that has not yet been answered concerns the relationship between feeding practices and overweight in infancy and childhood, and obesity in adulthood. Although no long-term prospective studies have been done, retrospective and short-term prospective studies tend to support the hypothesis of a close link.

Studies of the relationship between overweight at birth and obesity in childhood have generally shown a very low correlation (38). A higher correlation has been found, however between obesity at 12 months of age and later in life (39), while it has also been determined that cases of severe obesity at this age have a greater tendency to persist. One limitation of these studies is that they use as a basis for comparison situations prevailing at one point during infancy, for example at birth or at 12 months of age; there are many non-dietary factors, however, that may help to explain the situation at any given moment.

There is a better correlation between weight gain during infancy and overweight later in life (40). For example, a recent prospective study showed that, while breast-fed and artificially fed infants had similar growth patterns during the first three months, weight gain was greater for the artificially fed infants with a difference at one year of 410 g more in boys and 750 g in girls (41). Overfeeding is one of the main risks associated with bottle-feeding and too early complementary feeding.

Breast-fed infants appear to regulate their food intake in accordance with their needs (see Chapter 2). Once a mother assumes responsibility of the amount of food her child receives, overfeeding becomes a possibility. Undue concern about infant nutrition can contribute to overfeeding, particularly in societies where the image of a healthy baby is a plump one. The consequences later in life may be related either to the infant's excess weight or to the acquisition of undesirable eating habits, or both.

Hypertension. High sodium intake is certainly one of the principal factors in the etiology of essential hypertension. A direct relationship is not easy to prove because there also appear to be contributing genetic factors, which make some individuals more vulnerable than others. However, the relationship between high sodium intake and hypertension has been proved experimentally in rats. Of greatest concern are experimental data showing that sensitive rats with a high sodium intake only during the first six weeks of life still developed hypertension one year later (42).

Breast milk is low in sodium (about 15 mg/

100 ml or 6.5 mmol/1). However, an infant's sodium intake can drastically increase when complementary foods are introduced (see Table 4.1, part B), in particular when they are prepared according to the taste of a mother whose own salt intake is high. Although there are no data to show that early high sodium intake has the same consequences later in life for humans as have been demonstrated in experimental animals, it has been suggested that the taste for salt may be established with the introduction of foods other than breast milk. The maintenance of this habit may in turn have a cumulative effect that results in ill health many years later.

Experimental and epidemiological evidence indicates that potassium plays a protective role where high sodium intake related to hypertension is concerned (43). While most fresh fruits and vegetables are high in potassium, their processing for use as complementary foods may drastically reduce their value as a source of this mineral as well as vitamin C.

An association has also been found between hypertension and obesity, although they may be etiologically unrelated and observed independently. Early feeding practices may be a common factor creating food habits that favour the development of both conditions.

Arteriosclerosis. The role of dietary factors in the pathogenesis of arteriosclerosis and ischaemic heart disease, which are major health problems in industrialized countries and, increasingly, in developing countries, is no longer in doubt. The nutritional factors involved include diets high in energy and rich in cholesterol and saturated fats, but low in poly-unsaturated fats. High protein intake has also been found to be associated with these conditions, although diet is only contributory in otherwise predisposed individuals. The relationship between dietary factors and the development of the disease has been proved through both prospective and cross-sectional comparisons among different populations.

It is difficult to establish this link at the individual level, however, both because people respond differently to a diet rich in saturated fats and the fact that many other variables are involved. It would be still more difficult to establish a link between infant-feeding practices and a disease that manifests itself only some 30–40 years later. It has been shown, however, that infants in the upper centiles of lipid blood levels tend to maintain those same levels two years later (44). Thus, it only makes good sense to avoid, in complementary feeding, the same dietary excesses that have proved to be undesirable later in life.

Food allergy. There is evidence that prolonged breast-feeding and the timely introduction of carefully selected complementary foods contribute to the prevention of food allergies, particularly in predisposed infants (45). This is true not only in respect of cow's-milk allergy but also where other foods are concerned. Cow's-milk allergy is manifested clinically by gastrointestinal, dermatological or respiratory symptoms of varying severity, and even by anaphylactic shock.

Using sensitive immunological methods, it has been demonstrated that the majority of infants fed artificially with cow's-milk-based formulas do indeed react to the foreign proteins. However, since only a few infants show clinical manifestations, and usually only those with severe symptomatology are diagnosed as having cow's-milk allergy, it is very difficult to know the disease's real incidence. In industrialized countries, where the majority of infants in question received cow's-milk-based formulas since very early in life, various studies show an estimated prevalence of clinical manifestation of about 1% (46). In most instances, the condition can be prevented altogether by avoiding the use of cow's-milk preparations during the first months of life.

It has been shown that prolonged breast-feeding also has a protective value where allergies to other foods are concerned. For example, in a study of infants born of parents suffering from eczema, it was demonstrated that a significant reduction in the incidence of the disease could be achieved by feeding breast milk exclusively for at least three months and avoiding allergenic foods during the initial stages of complementary feeding (47). In another prospective study of children followed from birth to three years of age, it was shown that infants who were breast-fed for six months, particularly those with a family history of allergies, had a lower incidence of atopic diseases than those who were artificially fed. In the latter group, complementary feeding was started at three and a half months with cooked vegetables and fruits, cereals were introduced at five months, and meat and eggs were given at six; a more varied diet was given by nine months of age (45). A study of 135 exclusively breast-fed children of families with a history of atopic disease showed that giving no solid foods before six months greatly reduced the rates of eczema and food intolerance at 12 months; matched controls were children with similar family histories who received solids when 4–6 months of age. Relative rates for the study groups and controls were 35% vs. 14% for eczema, and 37% vs. 7% for food intolerance (48).

Résumé

Le développement physiologique du nourrisson et ses implications sur l'alimentation de complément

Durant la période intra-utérine le fœtus est alimenté par la circulation sanguine maternelle par l'intermédiaire du placenta. Le tractus gastro-intestinal et l'appareil rénal se développent progressivement mais ne sont pas fonctionnels. Après la naissance la croissance rapide du nourrisson entraîne une élévation proportionnelle des besoins nutritionnels, il faut donc que l'alimentation soit adaptée. La manière de nourrir l'enfant est conditionnée par son degré de maturité fonctionnelle, en particulier en ce qui concerne l'utilisation des nutriments, les mécanismes d'excrétion et la lutte contre les infections.

L'ingestion des aliments est limitée au début aux liquides grâce au réflexe de succion et à la configuration particulière du palais du nouveau-né et aussi à cause du réflexe lingual ou d'expulsion qui disparaît entre 4 et 6 mois. Plus tard, entre 6 et 9 mois apparaît la mastication qui facilite l'absorption d'aliments solides. Le processus de digestion des sucres se réalise dans la partie proximale de l'intestin grêle pendant les premiers mois de la vie. C'est là et non pas dans la bouche que les polysaccharides comme l'amidon sont attaqués; la sécrétion amylasique à ce niveau ne représente cependant que 10% de celle de l'adulte. Pendant les 3 premiers mois de la vie il n'y a pas de sécrétion d'amylase pancréatique.

Pour la digestion des protéines on sait que la sécrétion gastrique d'acide chlorhydrique et de pepsine existe chez le nouveau-né à terme mais à de basses concentrations. Les protéines sont principalement digérées dans le grêle où l'activité protéolytique est équivalente à celle de l'adulte. Néanmoins des apports protéiques élevés sont à déconseiller dans la mesure où un déséquilibre métabolique peut se produire au niveau du rein entraînant une acidose. La perméabilité particulière de la muqueuse intestinale du jeune enfant aux grosses molécules protéiques pourrait avoir des conséquences antigéniques qui expliqueraient certaines allergies au lait de vache.

Les graisses relaient le glucose comme source principale d'énergie après la naissance. La lipolyse préduodénale est assurée par les lipases linguales et elle est renforcée par la lipase du lait maternel. Il ne semble pas qu'il y ait de problème majeur avec les vitamines et les minéraux. Le lait maternel étant de ce point de vue particulièrement favorable pour l'absorption de la vitamine A et du fer entre autres. On ignore les mécanismes qui augmentent la biodisponibilité du fer dans le lait maternel mais on a constaté qu'elle diminuait lorsque l'on supplémentait la ration par des aliments d'origine végétale. La grande perméabilité de l'intestin à l'eau et aux électrolytes peut entraîner plus facilement des déséquilibres dangereux en cas d'hyperosmolarité du bol intestinal. La capacité fonctionnelle du rein augmente rapidement pendant les premiers mois de la vie mais elle est limitée chez le nouveau-né parce que la filtration glomérulaire et la capacité de concentration sont basses.

Besoins nutritionnels. Ils sont quantitativement et qualitativement différents de ceux des enfants plus âgés et des adultes. Durant le premier mois par exemple, ils sont en calories et en protéines 3 fois plus importants par kilogramme de poids que chez l'adulte. Cependant le lait maternel est l'aliment idéal pour les enfants jusqu'à 4 à 6 mois, sauf pour les nouveau-nés de très petit poids de naissance qui doivent être supplémentés en fer entre autres nutriments. Pour les enfants nourris avec des substituts du lait maternel la situation est différente. A titre indicatif des tables de composition de certains aliments de complément sont fournies. Les besoins en énergie sont difficiles à apprécier, les recommandations du comité d'experts FAO/OMS de 1971 sur les besoins en protéines et en énergie représentaient une estimation des besoins à 120 kcal/kg/j entre 0 et 3 mois diminuant régulièrement pour atteindre 105 kcal/kg/j entre 9 et 12 mois. Une consultation plus récente (FAO/OMS/UNU, 1981) partant des mêmes valeurs aboutit à des besoins nettement plus bas aux âges intermédiaires pour remonter sensiblement à 12 mois. Les différences constatées expliquent pourquoi dans des circonstances normales, le lait maternel seul couvre les besoins des nourrissons au moins pour les 4 premiers mois de la vie et souvent jusqu'au sixième.

Alimentation de complément et sevrage. Par sevrage il faut entendre le passage progressif du nourrisson du lait de sa mère au régime habituel de la famille. Aux environs de 6 mois les enfants doivent recevoir d'autres aliments et ils sont physiologiquement et fonctionnellement en mesure de les utiliser. Une diversification alimentaire trop précoce présente des risques à court terme: diminution de la production de lait chez la mère, mal compensée dans certains cas par la valeur nutritive du ''complément''; les céréales peuvent limiter l'absorption du fer du lait maternel; et le risque de maladies diarrhéiques augmente, en particulier dans les pays en développement. A beaucoup plus long terme les effets négatifs sur la santé peuvent se traduire par une morbidité d'origine nutritionnelle due aux modifications diététiques introduites durant le jeune âge intriquée avec la création d'habitudes alimentaires entraînant des pratiques diététiques néfastes. Le fait par exemple d'aimer les aliments salés à l'âge adulte pourrait être le résultat d'expériences acquises durant la petite enfance. Ainsi obésité, hypertension et artériosclérose semblent pouvoir être associées à ces situations. De même les allergies d'origine alimentaire peuvent être prévenues par un allaitement maternel prolongé comme certaines études l'ont démontré.

References

1. **Herbst, J.J.** Development of sucking and swallowing. In: Lebenthal, E., ed. *A textbook of gastroenterology and nutrition in infancy, Vol. 1.* New York, Raven Press, 1981, p. 102.
2. **Auricchio, S. et al.** Intestinal glycosidase activities in the human embryo, fetus, and newborn. *Pediatrics,* **35**: 944–954 (1965).
3. **Lebenthal, E. & Lee, P.C.** Development of functional response in human exocrine pancreas. *Pediatrics,* **66**: 556–560 (1980).
4. **Lebenthal, E. & Lee, P.C.** Glucoamylase and disaccharidase activities in normal subjects and in patients with mucosal injury of the small intestine. *J. pediatr.,* **97**: 389–393 (1980).
5. **Lilibridge, C.B. & Townes, P.L.** Physiologic deficiency of pancreatic amylase in infancy: a factor in iatrogenic diarrhea. *J. pediatr.,* **82**: 279–282 (1973).
6. **Lebenthal, E. et al.** Development of disaccharidase in premature, small-for-gestational-age and full-term infants. In: Lebenthal, E., ed. *A textbook of gastroenterology and nutrition in infancy, Vol. 1.* New York, Raven Press, 1981, p. 417.
7. **Agunod, M. et al.** Correlative study of hydrochloric acid, pepsin and intrinsic factor secretion in newborns and infants. *Am. j. dig. dis.,* **14**: 400–414 (1969).
8. **Deren, J.S.** Development of structure and function in the fetal and newborn stomach. *Am. j. clin. nutr.,* **24**: 144–159 (1971).
9. **Hadorn, B.** Developmental aspects of intraluminal protein digestion. In: Lebenthal, E., ed. *A textbook of gastroenterology and nutrition in infancy, Vol. 1.* New York, Raven Press, 1981, p. 368.
10. **Walker, W.A. et al.** Intestinal uptake of macromolecules: effect of oral immunization. *Science,* **177**: 608–610 (1972).
11. **Zoppi, G. et al.** Exocrine pancreas function in premature and full-term neonates. *Pediatr. res.,* **6**: 880–886 (1972).
12. **Poley, J.R. et al.** Bile acids in infants and children. *J. lab. clin. med.,* **63**: 838–846 (1964).
13. **Hamosh, M. & Burns, W.A.** Lipolytic activity of human

lingual glands (Ebner). *Lab. invest.*, **37**: 603–608 (1977).

14. **Hall, B. & Muller, D.P.R.** Studies on the bile salt stimulated lipolytic activity of human milk using whole milk as source of both substrate and enzyme. I. Nutritional implications. *Pediatr. res.*, **16**: 251–255 (1982).

15. **Weijers, H.A. et al.** Analysis and interpretation of the fat-absorption coefficient. *Acta pediatr. (Uppsala)*, **49**: 615–625 (1960).

16. **Saarinen, U.M. et al.** Iron absorption in infants: high bioavailability of breast-milk iron as indicated by the extrinsic tag method of iron absorption and by the concentration of serum ferritin. *J. pediatr.*, **91**: 36–39 (1977).

17. **Oski, F.A.** Development of the small intestine's capacity to absorb iron and folic acid. In: Lebenthal, E., ed. *Textbook of gastroenterology and nutrition in infancy, Vol. 1.* New York, Raven Press. 1981, p. 612.

18. **Aperia, A. et al.** Development of renal control of salt and fluid homeostasis during the first year of life. *Acta paediatr. scand.*, **64**: 393–398 (1975).

19. **Svenningsen, N.W. & Lindquist, B.** Postnatal development of renal hydrogen ion excretion capacity in relation to age and protein intake. *Acta paediatr. scand.*, **63**: 721–731 (1974).

20. **Oppe, T.E. et al.** Calcium and phosphorus levels in healthy newborn infants given various types of milk. *Lancet*, **1**: 1045–1048 (1968).

21. **Fomon, S.J. & Filer, L.J.** Amino acid requirements for normal growth. In: Nyhan, W.L., ed. *Amino acid metabolism and genetic variation.* New York, McGraw-Hill, 1967, p. 391.

22. WHO Technical Report Series No. 724, 1985 (*Energy and protein requirements*: report of a Joint FAO/WHO/UNU Expert Consultation), pp. 64–66.

23. WHO Technical Report Series No. 522, 1973 (*Energy and protein requirements*: report of a Joint FAO/WHO Ad Hoc Expert Committee).

24. **Fomon, S.J.** *Infant nutrition*, Philadelphia, Saunders, 1967.

25. FAO Nutritional Studies No. 15, 1957 (*Calorie requirements*: report of the Second Committee on Calorie Requirements).

26. **Waterlow, J.C. & Thomson, A.M.** Observations on the adequacy of breast-feeding. *Lancet*, **2**: 800–241 (1979).

27. WHO Technical Report Series No. 724 (see ref. *22*), *op. cit.*, pp. 90–92.

28. **Whitehead, R.G. et al.** A critical analysis of measured food intakes during infancy and early childhood in comparison with current international recommendations. *J. human nutr.*, **35**: 339–348 (1981).

29. **Habicht, J.P. et al.** Height and weight standards for preschool children. How relevant are ethnic differences in growth potential? *Lancet*, **1**: 611–614 (1974).

30. **Ahn, C.H. & Maclean Jr. W.C.** Growth of the exclusively breast-fed infant. *Am. j. clin. nutr.*, **33**: 183–192 (1980).

31. **Gordon, J.E. et al.** Weaning diarrhea, *Am. j. med. sci.*, **245**: 345–377 (1963).

32. **Black, R.E. et al.** Contamination of weaning foods and transmission of enterotoxigenic *Escherichia coli* diarrhoea in children in rural Bangladesh. *Trans. Roy. Soc. Trop. Med. Hyg.*, **76**: 259–264 (1982).

33. **Van Steenbergen, W.M. et al.** Agents affecting health of mother, infant and child in a rural area of Kenya. XXII. Bacterial contamination of foods commonly eaten by young children in Machakos, Kenya. *Trop. geogr. med.*, **35**: 193–197 (1983).

34. **Samadi, A.R., et al.** Detection of rotavirus in hand washing of attendants of children with diarrhoea. *Br. med. j.*, **286**: 188 (1983).

35. **Khan, M.V.** Interruption of shigellosis by hand-washing. *Trans. Roy. Soc. Trop. Med. Hyg.*, **76**: 164–168 (1982).

36. **Hebert, J.R.** Effects of water quality and water quantity on nutritional status: findings from a south Indian community. *Bull. Wld Hlth Org.*, **63**: 143–155 (1985).

37. **Jiwa. S. et al.** Enterotoxigenic bacteria in food and water from an Ethiopian community. *Appl. environ. microbiol.*, **41**: 1010–1019 (1981).

38. **Fisch, R.O. et al.** Obesity and leanness at birth and their relationship to body variations in later childhood. *Pediatrics*, **56**: 521–528 (1975).

39. **Johnston, F.E. & Marck, R.W.** Obesity in urban black adolescents of high and low relative weight at one year of age. *Am. j. dis. child.*, **132**: 862–864 (1978).

40. **Eid, E.E.** Follow-up study of physical growth of children who had excessive weight gain in first six months of life. *Br. med. j.*, **2**: 74–76 (1970).

41. **Hitchcock, N.E. et al.** The growth of breast-fed and artificially fed infants from birth to twelve months. *Acta paediatr. scand.*, **74**: 240–245 (1985).

42. **Dahl, L.K. et al.** Effects of chronic excess salt ingestion: evidence that genetic factors play an important role in susceptibility to experimental hypertension. *J. exp. med.*, **115**: 1173–1190 (1962).

43. **James, W.P.T.** Diseases of Western civilization. In: McLaren, D.S. & Burman, D., ed. *Textbook of paediatric nutrition, 2nd ed.* Edinburgh, Churchill Livingstone, 1982, p. 419.

44. **Mellies, M. & Glueck, C.** Infant feeding practices and the development of atherosclerosis. In: Lebenthal, E., ed. *Textbook of gastroenterology and nutrition in infancy, Vol. 2.* New York, Raven Press, 1981, p. 722.

45. **Saarinen, U.M. et al.** Prolonged breast-feeding as prophylaxis for atopic disease. *Lancet*, **2**: 163–166 (1979).

46. **Savilahti, E. et al.** Cow's-milk allergy. In: Lebenthal, E., ed. *Textbook of gastroenterology and nutrition in infancy, Vol. 2.* New York, Raven Press, 1981, p. 690.

47. **Matthew, D.J. et al.** Prevention of eczema. *Lancet*, **1**: 321–324 (1977).

48. **Kayosaari, M. & Saarinen, V.** Prophylaxis of atopic disease by six months' total solid food elimination. Evaluation of 135 exclusively breast-fed infants of atopic families. *Acta paediatr. scand.*, **72**: 411–414 (1983).

5. The low-birth-weight infant

Low-birth-weight (LBW) infants have special nutritional requirements arising from their rapid growth rate and developmental immaturity. LBW infants are of many kinds; for example, the nutritional needs and functional capabilities of a small-for-gestational-age full-term infant are not the same as those of a very LBW premature infant. Ideal criteria for evaluating the nutritional management of these infants have not been established, and thus the recommended intakes given here do not represent proven physiological requirements. They nevertheless provide a basis from which more refined recommendations may be made.

Although this chapter is not intended as such to be a discussion of applicable feeding techniques, it would be difficult and artificial to divorce two such closely intertwined aspects of the distinctive needs of this highly vulnerable group. Feeding techniques have to be carefully assessed in the light of specific environments and the expertise available, and none is entirely risk-free in any setting. Thus, it is essential to compensate for the immaturity of the infants and to avoid compromising the airway or risking aspiration of gastric contents.

The choice between using breast milk or proprietary formulas in feeding LBW infants is complex on both nutritional and immunological grounds as well as for practical reasons. Given that the preponderance (>90%) of LBW infants are born in developing countries, the use of an infant's own mother's fresh milk may be the only realistic option. However, irrespective of the health care facilities, level of technology or alternative formulas that might be available, studies show that there is much to recommend feeding LBW infants their own mothers' milk in any environment.

Introduction

Worldwide, about 16% of live births, or some 20 million infants per year, are of low birth weight (LBW: <2.5 kg) (*1*); these can be categorized further as very low birth weight (VLBW: <1.5–1.0 kg) and extremely low birth weight (ELBW: <1 kg). These infants, over 90% of whom are born in developing countries (*1*), have special nutritional requirements arising from their rapid fetal growth rate (15–20 g/kg/d at 24–36 weeks post-conceptional age) and developmental immaturity. The needs of the individual LBW infant vary widely, however; thus, for example, the nutritional requirements and functional capabilities of the small-for-gestational-age infant born at term are not the same as those of a premature infant, i.e., one born before 37 completed weeks of gestation (*2*), of the same birth weight.

Generally speaking, infants of 35 weeks gestational age or more, who constitute the great majority of premature infants, can and should receive breast milk. While breast milk may have to be supplemented for some of the smaller proportion of infants who are born between 32 and 35 weeks gestation, virtually all of them can be successfully breast-fed, or at least fed on breast milk. Infants of <32 weeks gestation, most of whom have birth weights <1500 g, form an exceptional group given their unusually high nutritional requirements. Initially, parenteral nutrition may be necessary for these infants, and its importance in specific circumstances should not be underestimated.

Developments in the nutritional management of the LBW infant have been reviewed (*3–5*) and recommendations published (*3–7*); these articles should be consulted for more detailed information. In particular, the report entitled "Nutrition and feeding of preterm infants" of the European Society of Paediatric Gastroenterology and Nutrition (ESP-GAN) provides a considered evaluation of recommendations; the report's main points are summarized below (*5*).

Ideal criteria for evaluating the nutritional management of LBW infants have not been established (*5*). Since metabolic demands after birth differ from those *in utero*, criteria based on intrauterine growth rates, body composition and factorial assessment of nutrient accretion are not ideal. Such extrapolations are unreliable not only because of the variable quality of the data on which they are based, but also because preterm infants, after delivery, rapidly lose extracellular fluid (ECF) and assume ECF:ICF (intracellular fluid) ratios similar to those of term infants. This 8–10% weight loss after delivery makes it unreliable to use the intrauterine nutrient accumulation as a reference for the LBW infant. Recommended intakes for some nutrients have been derived empirically by calculating the amount that would be supplied by breast milk.

The adequacy of nutrient supply can also be evaluated by monitoring biochemical consequences of supplying "idealized" nutrient requirements, but here again difficulties arise from not knowing if intrauterine or extrauterine biochemical values are suitable reference points. The solution to this problem will not emerge merely by avoiding short-term biochemical disasters. It also requires the systematic follow-up of LBW infants over the long term.

The recommended intakes given here do not represent proven physiological requirements for LBW infants. They nevertheless provide a basis from which more refined recommendations may be made.

Feeding techniques and related care

As with other chapters, the purpose of the present review is to describe the physiological characteristics of the infant and the resulting metabolic demands and recommended energy and nutrient intakes, based on the best available scientific evidence. It is not intended as such to be a discussion of applicable feeding techniques for this particular category of infant. Nevertheless, it would be both difficult and artificial to divorce entirely two such closely intertwined aspects of the distinctive needs of this highly vulnerable group of infants.

There are a number of underlying principles governing the feeding of LBW infants. First, feeding techniques (3–5) have to be carefully assessed in the light of the specific environment in which the infants in question are born. The use of a given technique clearly depends on the expertise available to those caring for the infants in question, and none is entirely risk-free in any setting.

The umbilical nutrition of the fetus has led some to argue simplistically that it would be desirable to feed all very immature infants in the first instance by a parenteral route. In this way the complications of enteral feeding such as aspiration pneumonia and necrotizing enterocolitis (a severe inflammation of the bowel in which parts of the bowel die of infection and have to be removed) may be avoided. But parenteral nutrition has its own complications such as systemic infection and metabolic imbalance and, in addition, is both costly and labour intensive. Parenteral feeding should be reserved for those preterm infants with medical or surgical gut problems that prevent enteral feeding for more than 3 days (8).

It is essential to compensate for the immaturity of LBW infants and to avoid compromising the airway or risking aspiration of gastric contents. During the initial phase of care, especially for VLBW and ELBW infants, neither oral nor intragastric feeding

may be tolerated or be practicable. These infants nevertheless still require energy, protein and carbohydrates to minimize catabolism of lean tissue and to prevent hypoglycaemia. Thus, an initial phase of total parenteral nutrition may be necessary and is favoured by many as an elective procedure. Older and more mature infants may, however, tolerate intragastric feeds. Critically ill infants, irrespective of whether they are being ventilated, are best managed with total parenteral nutrition, which should be maintained until they are either extubated or stable.

Although swallowing occurs *in utero* as early as 16 weeks gestation and elements of intestinal motility can be detected towards the end of the second trimester, organized oesophageal activity does not develop until about 34 weeks gestation when effective nutritional sucking can be sustained (9). In the LBW infant, at 28 weeks gestation, low antral pressures impair gastric emptying. Combined with lower oesophageal sphincter pressures, this may predispose the infant to oesophageal reflux.

Large enteral intakes may not be tolerated and injudicious persistence with these may predispose to reflux, regurgitation, gastric aspiration, apnoea, ileus, and necrotizing enterocolitis, especially if oesophago-gastrointestinal motility has not developed adequately. Furthermore, gastric capacity is limited in LBW infants and gastric distension may interfere with pulmonary function. Gastric emptying is faster with breast milk than with proprietary formulas, and can be improved by feeding the infant in the prone and lateral positions. Thus, in some LBW infants, optimum nutrition may only be achieved by a combination of enteral and parenteral techniques. In any event, even if parenteral nutrition is the dominant means of feeding, small amounts of some enteral feeds are beneficial because they create a more physiological endocrine response, stimulate bile flow and maintain maturation of the intestinal mucosa (8). Human milk has obvious additional advantages in this process. The wide range of hormones and growth factors, for example, may be particularly important for these infants (see chapter 2).

Even if infants can tolerate enteral feeding, feeds may still need to be given via indwelling tubes. The use of silastic tubes is probably preferable to using polyvinylchloride tubes since the silastic reduces the risk of intestinal perforation. The advantages of transpyloric over intragastric feeding are the subject of debate. Transpyloric feeding probably does not predispose to necrotizing enterocolitis, and placement of the tube in the duodenum rather than the jejunum avoids problems of impaired nutrient absorption, especially fats.

Similarly, the use of intermittent bolus or continuous infusion of feeds is controversial. The former is said to be more demanding of attendants' time, but continuous infusion does require constant monitoring to avoid gastric reflux. Intermittent enteral feeding would seem to be more physiological and recent studies indicate that adverse metabolic effects and altered body composition may arise from continuous feeding. These contrasts are probably caused by differences in the endocrine milieu.

The choice between using breast milk or proprietary formulas for LBW infants is a complex one. In addition to the nutritional and other implications of either feeding regimen for producing normal growth and development, however, there are the practical implications of whether or not these infants are able to suck.

It was demonstrated in a number of studies reported on a decade ago that LBW infants, some weighing even <1500 g at birth, can be breast-fed (10, 11). Success was attributed to such factors as highly motivated mothers who were permitted unrestricted access to their infants, an optimistic and knowledgeable nursing staff where attitudes towards breast-feeding were concerned, and the virtual absence of bottle-feeding in the health facilities in question. Manual or hand-pump expression of milk was used to the exclusion of mechanical pumps, and on occasion the mothers breast-fed other infants to stimulate milk secretion.

The first detailed clinical study of the effects of feeding undiluted breast milk very early to premature infants was reported in 1964 (12). The infants studied weighed between 1000 and 2000 g at birth and were fed with undiluted breast milk within 2 hours of birth in volumes of 60 ml/kg body weight given on the first day, increasing to 160 ml by the fourth day. This "early fed" group was compared with two other groups of low-birth-weight infants: (a) infants of comparable birth weight who were born during the study period but who were not fed until between 4 and 32 hours after delivery and given considerably less over the next week ("later fed"); and (b) infants weighing between 1000 and 2000 g who were born before the study period and who had been starved for at least 24 hours ("late-fed" infants). The results were impressive. The "early fed" infants regained their birth weight sooner and lost less weight than the other groups. Bilirubin levels were lower and there was also less symptomatic hypoglycaemia. There was no increase in the incidence of aspiration pneumonia.

Other studies have confirmed the benefits of early breast-feeding in reducing weight loss, raising blood glucose levels, and lowering unconjugated bilirubin in the serum. The first studies to show longer-term benefits of early feeding in 1968 reported that, at a mean age of 2 years, the intellectual and neurological development and physical growth of LBW infants who had been fed with breast milk early showed a considerable improvement over those children who were born at a time when delayed feeding was practised (13). This finding was confirmed a decade later when it was shown that early feeding is associated with higher blood sugar, lower bilirubin, less dehydration, and more rapid return to birth weight in the "early" than in the "late" group (14).

A more recent study (15) in England investigated the association in 771 LBW infants between a mother's choice to provide breast milk for her infant and her child's developmental status at 18 months postpartum. The breast-milk-fed group had significantly higher mental scale scores, even after adjusting for social and demographic influences. Whether this residual developmental advantage relates to parental factors, including the level of concern for an infant's welfare and perception of maternal role of a mother who decides to provide her own milk, or to a beneficial effect of human milk itself on brain development has important implications for the nutritional management of premature infants.

In the early 1980s, it was demonstrated that LBW infants fed human milk gained weight at roughly the same rate as infants fed formulas providing a protein intake of at least 2.25 g/kg/day (see below) and, also, that they did not develop some of the metabolic abnormalities observed in formula-fed infants (16). More recently, clinical studies have shown that infants fed their own mothers' milk have superior rates of weight gain than infants fed donor milk; this is due to the higher levels of protein (approximately 30%) (17) and sodium, chloride, magnesium and iron (18) in the milk of mothers who deliver prematurely than in the milk of mothers who deliver at term. The nutrients supplied to a 33-week preterm infant fed 200 ml/kg/d of "average" preterm milk were in excess of calculated intrauterine requirements for protein and minerals except calcium, phosphorus and iron (18). Thus, while hyponatraemia is uncommon in prematurely born infants fed their own mothers' milk, skeletal mineralization of these infants is suboptimal (16). Moreover, it is questionable whether human milk contains sufficient vitamin D for the requirements of these infants (19).

On both practical and economic grounds, however, the use of the infant's own mother's fresh milk may be essential, especially in view of the fact that the preponderance of LBW deliveries occurs in developing countries (1). Even though such milk, compared with full-term mothers' milk, may be disadvantageous because of its variable and unpredictable nutrient content, it still presents the many advantages that human milk in the raw state has over artificial formulas (see chapter 2). These advantages may in turn outweigh any disadvantages that arise from the uncertainty of knowing an infant's precise nutrient intake, and the attendant risk of undernutrition, particularly as regards energy, water, sodium, calcium and phosphorus, zinc, vitamin C, and folic acid. In any case, awareness of these risks permits monitoring for manifestations and correction of any deficiency by supplementing breast milk in culturally appropriate ways.

In Finland, where proprietary formulas have never gained widespread acceptance in the feeding of premature infants, human milk has been in almost continuous use. Thus, human milk banking has been carried out on a relatively large scale; about 5000 litres per million individuals are collected annually and used for this purpose (20). About half of the mothers who deliver VLBW infants of < 1500 g at birth are able to lactate enough so that the infants can be fed with their own mothers' milk (20).

Feeding VLBW infants on human milk supplemented with human milk protein has been shown to lead to improved serum total protein and blood haemoglobin concentrations during the second month of life (21). A study in Finland evaluating the effect of added human milk protein on the growth of human-milk-fed VLBW infants during the first few weeks of life concluded that protein supplementation improves the growth of small premature infants fed human milk, and that the protein concentration of bank milk is insufficient for their adequate growth (22).

The practice in the Royal Children's Hospital in Melbourne, Australia, is to use each mother's own expressed breast milk, whenever possible, to feed VLBW infants. With relatively simple techniques, mothers can produce milk consistently with minimal bacterial contamination, although infants grow more slowly than those fed on specialized formulas (23).

Motivated initially by sheer economic necessity, neonatal units in a number of developing countries have begun to adopt, with encouraging results, the exclusive use of preterm breast milk combined with simple interventions to meet the special needs of LBW infants. For example, the results of a recent study (24) in India (Kota), where 30–40% of all births are LBW (25), are of particular importance given their implications for the application of economical and nutritionally adequate technology in developing countries. The study sought to provide adequate calories for optimal growth in 21 LBW infants between 1.0 and 1.75 kg and gestational age 28–35 weeks by fortifying fresh preterm human milk with medium-chained triglycerides (MCT) (coconut oil) and sucrose. No infant in the study had symptoms of diarrhoea and vomiting, nor did any develop necrotizing enterocolitis. Feeding the fortified formula (MCT + sugar + preterm milk + vitamins +

iron), which was done initially by intermittent gavage and later by small spoon/dropper, was sufficient to achieve postnatal gains in weight and height similar to intrauterine rates. It seemed unnecessary to add extra protein. Long-term achievement of motor and mental milestones was normal in 90% of the infants, who were followed for a total of 10–12 months.

In one hospital in Bombay, emphasis is placed on having mothers participate in the care of their babies and engaging in minimum handling and minimum interventions. Supportive aspects of this care include:

— exclusive human-milk feeding;
— establishing a "warm-chain" starting from the labour room to support the infant's temperature regulation;
— stabilizing nursery admissions by rapid re-warming and oxygenation to break the vicious cycle of hypothermia, hypoxaemia and hypoglycaemia;
— establishing perinatal audit sessions;
— developing management schedules for common problems like respiratory distress and asphyxia;
— teaching and training nurses and midwives in both the neonatal unit and the labour ward;
— utilizing the postnatal care ward as an intermediate care unit.

This approach led to a significant decline in the mortality rates for the three categories of infants (< 1250 g, 1251–1500 g and > 1500 g) as well as in total mortality; a shift in the periodicity of diarrhoeal episodes from endemicity to self-limiting episodes; and a reduction in health care expenditure. Follow-up of discharged babies showed that the post-neonatal mortality in this high-risk group was less than that for the general population in the city of Bombay, possibly as a result of the fact that few mothers had given up breast-feeding by one year postpartum (26).

The Kenyatta National Hospital and Pumwani Maternity Hospital in Nairobi both have special care units for sick infants and those weighing < 2000 g; many are in the VLBW category (< 1500 g) (27). Mothers lodge in nearby dormitories and come to the units every 3 hours, day and night, where they hand-express milk into sterilized containers. The milk volumes thus produced are usually adequate for the infants' needs. Mothers are actively engaged in the care of their infants; skin-to-skin contact is encouraged even before the infants are ready to suck. Until infants can swallow, nurses feed the mothers' own freshly expressed milk by gavage, adding calcium and other nutrients when necessary. When infants reach about 1600 g, their mothers take over, giving a measured quantity of their milk by cup, which is sterilized. No bottles are used in either unit. Direct *ad libitum* breast-feeding begins when the infants' weight reaches about 1700 g. Exclusive use of the mothers' own fresh milk has dramatically lessened neonatal diarrhoea and other infections. Most infants are discharged fully breast-fed before they weigh 2000 g.

Feeding the LBW infant directly from the breast has distinct advantages. For example, one set of studies has examined infants who were fed their own mothers' milk either directly or from a bottle: with breast-feeding, the infant's temperature and oxygenation remained stable; with bottle-feeding, and for some minutes thereafter, the temperature and blood oxygen levels fell significantly (28).

The above examples and others in Helsinki, Manila, Oslo and Stockholm (see chapter 2 on the particular importance for the premature and LBW infant of breast milk's immunological qualities) offer important insights into the nutritional management of this highly vulnerable category of infant. They also demonstrate that, irrespective of the health care facilities, level of technology or alternative formulas that might be available, there is much to recommend this feeding regimen (29) in both developed and developing countries. Finally, this approach presents the added advantage of involving mothers directly in the care of their infants, while at the same time helping to establish lactation.

Recommended intakes for LBW infants

The optimal diet for the LBW infant is still to be defined (30). As noted above, the recommended intakes that follow do not represent proven physiological requirements for LBW infants. They nevertheless provide a basis from which more refined recommendations may be made.

Water

At between 26 and 36 weeks gestation, water constitutes 70–80% of fetal weight gain. Postpartum, irrespective of gestational age, this ratio falls to 50–70%. Thus, of a weight gain of 20 g, 12 g (ml) is water. This is a small amount compared to water losses, which are the principal determinants of water requirements.

Water is lost through renal and extrarenal routes. Of the extrarenal loss, insensible water loss (IWL) via the skin (transepidermal water loss, TEWL) and lungs amounts to 30–60 ml daily. IWL is increased by activity, respiratory stress, and low ambient humidity and/or high temperature. After 32 weeks gestation, TEWL in the first 3 days of life can amount to 2–6 ml/kg/h (8 g/m²/h); however, losses are much higher in infants with shorter gestations (31, 32). Since the epidermis matures rapidly indepen-

dently of gestation, TEWL at 1–2 weeks of postnatal age is similar to that of term infants. Nursing under radiant heaters and phototherapy can increase TEWL by 2–3-fold and 50%, respectively, and will consequently increase the water requirements. Early water loss can be reduced by keeping LBW infants wrapped and in an air humidity of 80% or more; nursing with a heat shield can increase local humidity and reduce TEWL by 30%. Respiratory water loss is increased if infants are ventilated with unhumidified air. Fecal water loss is between 5 and 20 ml/kg body weight daily.

Urinary volume depends on the osmotic load which is excreted. Even with maximum arginine-vasopressin (antidiuretic hormone, ADH) stimulation, neonates cannot achieve a urinary osmolality greater than 500 mosm/kg; more usually, it is 60–200 mosm/kg (10). Thus, assuming that most LBW infants can achieve a urinary osmolality of 170 mosm/kg, the customary renal solute load (14–15 mosm/kg body weight daily) would be excreted in 90 ml/kg/d. Summing these losses indicates a daily water requirement of 150–200 ml/kg body weight. Some of this requirement is produced endogenously by nutrient oxidation (approximately 12 ml/100 kcal), and thus based on a daily energy intake of 120–130 kcal/kg, 15 ml of water would be produced.

The practice has evolved of providing LBW neonates, during the first week of life, with increasing volumes of water at 60, 90, 120 and 180 (150–200) ml/kg/d. The infants are able to tolerate intakes of 90–260 ml/kg/d from 3 days of age (33). The adequacy of their water intake should be monitored by clinical evaluation, regular weighing, determination of plasma sodium, and by measuring urine specific gravity or osmolality. IWL should be kept to a minimum and the increased requirements arising from clinical and nursing techniques should always be borne in mind. Inappropriate secretion of AVP induced during stress, for example asphyxia or respiratory distress, may reduce urine volume and cause water overloading (34). This may require water restriction but the coincident risk of restricting the intakes of other nutrients should not be overlooked.

Energy

Energy (3, 5) is expended in the resting metabolic rate and as a result of activity, thermal regulation, tissue synthesis and dermal evaporative water loss; it is stored in newly synthesized tissue and is lost in faeces and urine.

LBW infants, irrespective of their size relative to gestation, require relatively higher energy intakes than heavier or term infants because they have higher resting metabolic rates, inefficient intestinal absorption, less efficient thermal regulation and increased growth rates (35). The resting metabolic rate requires 36–60 kcal/kg/d; it increases during the neonatal period and is higher in infants who are small for date than in those who have grown appropriately, who are on high energy intakes, or who are growing fast or recovering from starvation.

The energy cost of growth comprises that needed for the synthesis of new tissues and the energy which is deposited in them. Estimates of the cost of tissue synthesis vary considerably with the composition and hydration of the new tissue, rates of growth and the supply of other nutrients, for example protein, essential amino acids, Mg and Zn, which are needed for efficient growth and lean-tissue synthesis. Generally speaking, the energy cost of growth is 5 kcal/g (range 3.0–5.7) (3, 5, 35, 36). On this basis, at a representative weight gain of 15 g/kg/d, and allowing for tissue water content, the energy requirement for synthesis would be 10–25 kcal, and the energy stored in the tissue would be 20–30 kcal.

The energy intake lost in faeces varies with the efficiency of intestinal absorption and with dietary composition. Optimal absorption of energy can be achieved by paying special attention to the quality and quantity of fat (see below) and carbohydrate constituents. Under ideal conditions, an absorptive efficiency of 80% or more can be expected in the stable LBW infant, resulting in a daily faecal loss of 10–30 kcal/kg (35). Energy used in spontaneous activity and crying is between 5–10 kcal/kg/d.

Evaporative water loss increases energy requirements but these can be reduced by measures that minimize IWL. The energy required for thermoregulation can be minimized by paying scrupulous attention to maintaining the child in a thermoneutral environment and by avoiding cooling during nursing procedures. Infants maintained just below their thermoneutral environment lose 7–8 kcal/kg/d; in a cool or temperate climate it thus seems wise to allow up to 10 kcal/kg/d for thermoregulatory activity.

Daily intakes of 95–165 kcal/kg would be needed to match the losses outlined above; the upper limit is probably an overestimate but it is currently thought to be most appropriate to meet a recommended requirement of 120–130 kcal/kg/d (3, 5, 35). Since human breast milk has an energy density of 65–70 kcal/dl, this energy requirement could be met with a volume of 180–200 ml/kg/d. There is no clear evidence that the energy density of milk from mothers who deliver preterm is higher than that from mothers delivering at term. Proprietary formulas with an energy density of 65–85 kcal/dl will meet these requirements at volumes of 200–150 ml/kg/d. Pasteurized breast milk does not support growth as well as raw breast milk. There is probably no benefit in providing higher energy intakes; the LBW baby

just becomes fat. Although small-for-gestational age LBW infants grow faster than those of appropriate size for date, they do this with a lower energy (fat) deposition and higher water deposition in tissue (37) and do not necessarily benefit from increased energy intakes.

Protein (3–5)

Approximately 90% of absorbed dietary protein nitrogen is incorporated in infants' tissues but this operation's efficiency and the level of tolerance of dietary protein depend on the quality of the protein, the availability of energy and other nutrients (for example Mg, Zn, P) which ensure its efficient use, and the maturation of amino-acid metabolism and renal excretory mechanisms.

The nitrogen content of the fetus rises from 14.6 g/kg at 24 weeks gestation to 18.6 g/kg at 36 weeks gestation; the respective nitrogen accretion rates are 252 mg/kg/d and 320 mg/kg/d (38). Multiplying these figures by 6.25 to derive an estimate of daily net protein accumulation gives corresponding figures of 1.6 g and 2.0 g/kg. Glycine, cysteine and taurine may be essential amino acids in the LBW infant because of an increased requirement and the immaturity of their endogenous synthetic pathways.

As a rule of thumb, protein should comprise about 10% of energy intake. Inappropriately high intakes (>4 g/kg/d), impaired utilization of amino acids and proteins that is secondary to deficiencies of other nutrients, and stress and infections all predispose to protein catabolism, acidosis, hyperammonaemia, raised blood urea, and increased renal solute load. The delicacy of these interrelationships demonstrates the biochemical vulnerability of LBW infants. Even stable LBW infants, especially those who are on high protein intakes, are susceptible to developing high plasma concentrations of phenylalanine, tyrosine and methionine; this is probably secondary to immature activities of parahydroxyphenyl pyruvic acid hydrolase and cystathionase.

Protein requirements of LBW infants are calculated to be 2.9 and 3.5 g/kg/d at 24 and 36 weeks, respectively. These intakes approximate 2.2 and 2.7 g/ 100 kcal in a feed providing 130 kcal/kg/d. It has been suggested that an infant formula should provide at least 2.25 g/100 kcal, that is 2.9 g/kg/d at an intake of 130 kcal/kg. Protein intakes greater than 4 g/kg/d (3.1 g/100 kcal) may not be used effectively (39) and should be avoided.

Early breast milk contains about 25 g of protein per litre. By the time lactation is established this falls to a nitrogen equivalent of about 12 g of protein per litre; of this, 25% is in the form of non-protein nitrogen as urea and nucleotides. Furthermore, not all the protein may be absorbed; secretory IgA (10%

of the total protein present), lactoferrin and lysozyme may be excreted intact in the faeces. Thus the effective available protein in breast milk is about 7 g/l.

The metabolic significance of the non-protein nitrogenous compounds is a fascinating and unresolved problem. The protein in raw breast milk is better utilized than that in infant formula. None the less, even on daily intakes of 180–200 ml/kg of breast milk, infants may still not receive adequate protein, especially if they are gaining weight rapidly and supplementation with breast-milk protein (40) or with hydrolysed casein (41) is being evaluated.

Considering all these points, it has been recommended that proprietary cow's-milk-based formulas should be whey predominant and should contain 1.8–2.4 g of protein per dl at 2.2–3.2 g/100 kcal, which would provide 2.9–4.0 g/kg/d. The protein content of breast milk may not match these recommended intakes, and thus the practice has developed of supplementing breast milk for LBW infants with a whey formula or, more occasionally, human-milk protein (40) (see examples above).

Taurine (42)

This sulphur beta amino acid may be a growth factor. Preterm infants have low plasma and urinary concentrations of taurine, which may represent a relative inefficiency of the rate-limiting synthetic enzyme cysteine-sulphonic acid decarboxylase. Taurine supplements in some LBW infants on parenteral nutrition increased the plasma taurine acid concentrations and normalized the electroretinograms. However, the case for routine supplementation is not universally recognized, even if it has been accepted that most proprietary formulas should be fortified to match the taurine content of breast milk (about 5 mg/dl).

Fat (5)

Fat provides 50% of the energy in breast milk, irrespective of whether the milk is from mothers who delivered before or at term. Reduced secretion of pancreatic lipase and low intraluminal bile-salt concentrations limit the intestinal absorption of lipids in preterm infants even more than in those infants born at term. Fat constitutes 1% of body weight at 26 weeks gestation and 16% at term, representing an accumulation of about 550 g during the last 14 weeks of gestation.

Breast milk contains higher amounts of long-chain unsaturated fatty acids (linoleic (C18:2w6), linolenic (C18:3w3), arachidonic (C20:4w6) and docosahexanoic (C22:6w3)) than cow's milk lipid in which palmitic acid (C16:0) is the predominant fatty acid. Unsaturated fatty acids are more efficiently absorbed than are saturated fatty acids of the same chain length; in breast milk 60–70% of the long-chain fatty acids are unsaturated, whereas approximately 60% of those in cow's milk are saturated. The role of the polyenoic acids in breast milk is unknown but they accumulate rapidly in the fetal brain during the last trimester of pregnancy (43).

The fatty acids in the 2 (beta) position in triacylglycerols are less readily hydrolysed by pancreatic lipase than those in the 1 and 3 positions. In breast milk over 95% of the lipid is triacylglycerol; in this case the predominant beta ester is palmitic acid. The resultant product of hydrolysis, palmitate monoacylglycerol, is well absorbed. In contrast, palmitate is a less well absorbed form in cow's milk lipid because only about 30% is esterified to the beta position of glycerol.

Because the milk of all mothers, including those who give birth to LBW infants, has a variable fat content during the course of a single feeding (see chapter 2), LBW infants should not be fed solely on foremilk. This was underscored by a recent study which examined the growth rate of one group of infants fed with pooled drip milk, which is known to be low in fat, and another group fed on a high-calorie experimental formula. There was no control group of infants fed on breast milk having a balanced fat composition. Growth outcomes were better for the infants fed on the experimental formula (44).

LBW infants have clinical, biochemical and histological evidence of essential fatty acid deficiency if their linoleic-acid intake comprises less than 1% of their energy intake. Consequently, it has been suggested that in proprietary formulas linoleic acid should account for at least 4.5% of total calories (that is, 0.5 g/100 kcal), and that linolenic acid should provide at least 0.5% of total calories (55 mg/100 kcal).

Since there are clear advantages to having unsaturated fatty acids in infant feeds, many proprietary formulas are now prepared using vegetable oils. Measures that improve the efficiency of fat absorption also improve the utilization of energy, minerals (for example Ca, Mg, and Zn), and nitrogen.

Medium-chain fatty acids (MCFA; C8–12) are more easily absorbed than long-chain fatty acids and can enter the mitochondria for oxidation without the carnitine transfer system. For these reasons, and because milk of mothers of preterm infants has 2–3 times more MCFA than does full-term mothers' milk, MCFA have been used in feeding LBW babies. The use of medium-chain triglycerides (MCT) in infant formula results in up to a 20% improvement in absorption efficiency. This has not been associated with significantly better energy balances or weight gains, although these may in fact be inappropriate outcomes to monitor. MCT and their constituent fatty acids become incorporated in adipose tissues and membranes, but no adverse effects have been seen in infants fed formulas containing up to 80% of fat as MCT.

The ESPGAN Nutrition Committee has recommended that formulas should not contain more than 40% of fat as MCT. In quantitative terms, at an energy intake of 130 kcal/kg/d and a maximum recommended carbohydrate and protein intake, the recommended fat intake would be 4.7 g/kg (3.6 g/100 kcal). The suggested intake range is 4–9 g/kg/d (with a maximum lipid density in formula of 7 g/100 kcal).

Carnitine (5)

Carnitine (beta-hydroxy-gamma-tricthylamino butyric acid), a quaternary amino acid, is essential for fatty-acid oxidation because it transports long-chain fatty acids across the inner mitochondrial membrane. Reduced plasma and tissue concentrations of carnitine in some preterm infants suggest that their endogenous synthesis of carnitine is reduced, but no deficiency syndrome has been detected and there is, as yet, no case for supplementation. Since breast milk contains 39–63 μmol/l, it has been proposed that proprietary formulas be supplemented to provide at least 60–90 μmol/l.

Carbohydrate

Intestinal disaccharidase activities are present from 14 weeks of gestation. At mid-gestation the activities of lactase, sucrase, isomaltase and maltase are approximately 70–50% of those at term and clinical experience shows that preterm infants tolerate the corresponding disaccharides well. Although lactose is not essential (its constituent, galactose, which is needed for cerebroside and glycosaminoglycan synthesis, can be derived from glucose in the liver), there is a case for providing carbohydrate in this form for non-breast-fed preterm infants because it enhances the intestinal absorption of minerals and promotes the growth of intestinal lactobacilli. The intraluminal hydrolysis of the short-chain polysaccharides present in breast milk is facilitated by endogenous alpha-amylase and by breast-milk alpha-amylase. However, the former may not be well developed in preterm infants, and may limit its use to reduce the osmolality of glucose polymers and partially hydrolysed starch as energy sources in formula.

The inclusion of sucrose in proprietary formulas is not associated with any demonstrable metabolic disadvantage, although it induces a higher insulin response than does lactose. Starch hydrolysates (for example corn-syrup solids and maltodextrins) are other possible carbohydrate sources.

Glucogenic pathways are established in preterm infants but they are less efficient and their function may be limited by the availability of substrates. The glucose requirement of LBW infants is higher than for term infants. Their respective glucose turnover rates are 5–6 mg/kg per minute and 3–5 mg/kg per minute (45). Since glucose is the main oxidative substrate for the brain, the LBW infant is vulnerable to hypoglycaemia. Since even moderate hypoglycaemia (that is, plasma glucose <2.6 mmol/l) can be associated with subsequent impaired neurodevelopment (46), every effort should be made to avoid its occurrence.

Breast milk contains about 7–8 g of lactose per dl (7.7 g/100 kcal) and requires no supplementation. A proposed lactose content of proprietary formulas is 3.2–12 g/100 kcal, not exceeding 8 g/dl. The total carbohydrate content recommended for such feeds is 7–14 g/100 kcal, with a maximum of 11 g/dl. Higher intakes could be used but they may cause osmotic diarrhoea and distort energy:protein ratios.

Minerals

Calcium and phosphorus (3–5). At 26–36 weeks gestation the fetus accumulates 120–150 mg of calcium per kg/d (3–3.25 mmol) and 60–75 mg (1.94–2.42 mmol) of phosphorus per kg/d. A 1-kg fetus has 5.7 g of calcium and 3.4 g of phosphorus, 99% and 80% of which, respectively, are found in the skeleton, the rest in the soft tissues. Neither breast milk nor proprietary formulas can match the calculated accretion rates for these minerals, which present the greatest problems for infants of less than 34 weeks post-conceptional age.

Early neonatal calcium deficiency may cause asymptomatic hypocalcaemia, which stimulates a release of parathormone and mobilization of skeletal calcium. Early introduction of feeds or of calcium with parenteral nutrition reduces this problem's incidence. Late neonatal hypocalcaemia (at 3–15 days of age), unless it is detected biochemically, can initially manifest itself by convulsions.

After birth, extensive bone turnover and remodelling, combined with continued bone growth, lead to reduced bone density, which is sometimes described as a "physiological osteoporosis". The range of bone changes can vary from a barely discernible radiological hypomineralization to severe rickets with fractures. The assessment of bone mineralization is difficult (47). Parameters that have been used to assess both this and calcium metabolism include calcium balances; biochemical indices of bone and calcium metabolism, for example plasma alkaline phosphatase activity; plasma concentrations of parathormone, calcium and phosphorus; radiological density; postmortem analysis; and photon densitometry.

This last technique may prove particularly useful in future, especially when combined with biochemical monitoring of systemic calcium and phosphorus homeostasis. As many as 57% of infants weighing < 1 kg may develop frank rickets (48). Nearly all infants < 1.5 kg in weight will develop reduced bone mineralization because they have impaired calcium retention irrespective of their calcium intake. Adequate deposition of skeletal calcium depends on the supply of phosphorus. These two minerals may well be the principal, though not the only, determinants of the development of metabolic bone disease (49, 50), although vitamin D deficiency may also play a role. Even high intakes of vitamin D, generating normal or raised plasma concentrations of vitamin D metabolites, do not necessarily prevent metabolic bone disease (50).

A phosphorus-depletion syndrome can develop in breast-fed LBW infants. The requirements for phosphorus retention can be calculated by using the following formula, which makes specific allowance for the phosphorus required for soft tissue synthesis:

$$\text{Phosphorus retention (mg)} = \frac{\text{calcium retention}}{2} + \frac{\text{nitrogen retention}}{17.4}$$

If these requirements, which approximate 0.6 mmol/kg/d, are not met by dietary intake, there is insufficient phosphorus available to maintain plasma inorganic phosphate, which falls below 1.5 mmol/l, and to incorporate calcium into bone. Thus, the phosphate-depletion syndrome is associated with elevated plasma calcium concentrations, hypercalciuria (> 0.4 mmol/kg/d), hypophosphaturia (< 0.1 mmol/kg/d), and an elevated plasma alkaline phosphatase activity (often above 1000 IU/l). Although this alteration in alkaline phosphatase activity has no specific prognostic value for individual patients, groups that have experienced such elevations during the neonatal period and infancy are ultimately shorter than those that have not.

Phosphate supplements (0.3 mmol/kg/d) improve calcium retention and eliminate hypercalciuria (51), but large phosphorus supplements may cause phosphaturia, hypocalcaemia and hypercalciuria (52). Growth is improved but hypomineralization is not prevented. The phosphate-depletion syndrome is rare in formula-fed LBW infants because their phosphorus intake is higher than that of breast-fed infants.

Calcium and phosphorus supplies should thus be carefully balanced. Calcium cannot be utilized effectively for bone formation in the absence of phosphorus and there is no evidence that calcium intakes > 140 mg/kg/d are effective in improving bone mineralization. Indeed, such intakes may be detrimental because they may lead to impaired fat absorption, intraluminal calcium precipitation, hypercalcaemia, metabolic acidosis and phosphorus depletion.

The calcium and phosphorus content of breast milk from mothers delivering preterm is 25–34 mg/l (0.62–0.85 mmol/l) and 11.6 mg/l (0.37 mmol/l), respectively, which is similar to that in term milk.

The ESPGAN Committee recommends that the range for calcium supplied by proprietary formulas be 1.75–3.5 mmol/100 kcal and that for phosphorus 1.6–2.9 mmol/100 kcal. In order to achieve optimum utilization of both minerals, the ideal calcium:phosphorus ratios are considered to be 1.4–2.0:1.0.

When calcium intake is low, particularly with LBW infants, the ratio of phosphorus to calcium should be high in order to provide for soft-tissue synthesis; this can be deduced from the above equation and, similarly, when calcium intake is low, lower Ca:P ratios are tolerated.

Magnesium (5). A 1-kg fetus has 0.2 g of magnesium; this increases to 0.8 g, 65% of which is in the skeleton, in the full-term infant weighing 3.5 kg. After potassium, magnesium is the major intracellular cation. It is essential for adequate protein and soft-tissue synthesis.

Hypomagnesaemia in preterm infants manifests itself by convulsions and persistent hypocalcaemia and may be associated with rapid weight gain. Factorial approaches suggest that at 1 kg the LBW infant should be accumulating 10 mg of magnesium per kg/d, while at 1.5 kg the rate is 8.5 mg/kg/d. Breast milk provides 3.0 mg/dl. It has been suggested that formulas for preterm infants should contain 6–12 mg of magnesium per 100 kcal (0.25–0.5 mmol/100 kcal).

Sodium (3–5). The 25-week fetus has 94 mmol of sodium per kg of body weight. By term, this has fallen to 74 mmol/kg. The daily accumulation of sodium in the second half of gestation is 0.5–1.1 mmol/kg.

In the first 4–5 days of life, the LBW infant loses about 12% of body weight and 6–16 mmol of sodium per kg. This loss occurs in spite of nitrogen and potassium retention and is independent of sodium intakes of 1–6 mmol/kg/d. Some 70–80% of the weight loss seen in infants weighing about 1 kg at birth is due to isotonic loss of ECF. Thus, the LBW infant assumes postnatally the ECF:ICF ratio of the term baby and the ECF loss is not regained. The most probable cause of hyponatraemia during the first 5 days of life is water retention secondary to inappropriate secretion of arginine-vasopressin (antidiuretic hormone, ADH).

Most LBW infants achieve positive sodium balance during the second week of life; intakes of 1.6 mmol sodium per kg/d can achieve this but do not necessarily prevent hyponatraemia (<130 mmol Na/l). On such intakes of sodium, some 50% of infants fed pooled breast milk and 20% of those fed proprietary formulas may develop late hyponatraemia. However, this can be corrected with intakes of 33 mmol Na/d. Infants, especially those under 30 weeks gestation with immature renal tubular sodium re-absorption, may need as much as 8–12 mmol/kg/d; the sodium intake can be adjusted to maintain normal plasma sodium concentrations (130–135 mmol/l) as the renal function matures. After 32–34 weeks of gestation LBW infants have lower sodium requirements; most are able to maintain normal plasma concentrations irrespective of whether they are fed a formula intended for full-term infants that provides 1.2 mmol/kg/d, or one for preterm infants providing 3.9 mmol/kg/d.

Since mature breast milk contains only 6.5 mmol Na/l, it may not provide sufficient sodium for growth and maintenance of plasma sodium concentrations in LBW term infants even when they are fed 200 ml/kg/d. It is therefore necessary to monitor continually plasma sodium concentrations, and sodium supplements in the form of sodium chloride (approximately 2–4 mmol/kg/d) should be provided when necessary. Infants fed their own mother's milk may be at a lower risk of hyponatraemia because such preterm milk can contain more sodium. However, because the content is variable, it is still necessary to monitor plasma sodium concentrations.

Since requirements vary so much with postnatal and post-conceptional ages, it is difficult to provide optimal sodium intakes for all LBW infants from a single formula. It has been recommended that the sodium content of proprietary formulas for preterm and LBW infants should be similar to those prepared for full-term babies. This would be in the range of 6.5–15 mmol Na/l (1.0–2.3 mmol/100 kcal), and thus ensure an overall intake of not less than 1.3 mmol/kg/d. Additional supplements can be given when appropriate.

Potassium (5). Potassium deficiency is rare, even during periods of rapid growth, and intakes matching those provided by breast milk would meet the needs of all LBW neonates. Thus, at concentrations of 10–17.5 mmol/l (1.5–2.6 mmol/100 kcal), a daily intake of 2.0–3.5 mmol/kg would be achieved. On this basis,

the potassium content of most formulas for preterm infants (15–25 mmol/l) is adequate for the LBW infant.

Chloride (4, 5). Chloride is the major anion in the ECF and, with sodium, contributes 80% of ECF oncotic activity. At 25 weeks gestation (500 g body weight), the chloride content of the human fetus is 70 mmol/kg, falling to 46 mmol/kg in the term (3.5 kg) infant. The daily accumulation of chloride is thus calculated as being 0.7 mmol/kg/d.

Dietary chloride deficiency has not been described in LBW infants, but it has developed in full-term infants fed soya-based or cow's-milk formula containing less than 3 mmol/l. Features included a failure to thrive, muscular weakness and hypotonia, vomiting and dehydration, anorexia, low plasma-chloride concentrations, hyponatraemia, hypokalaemia, hypocalcaemia and a metabolic alkalosis. The urine had a negligible chloride content.

As a routine precaution, therefore, low chloride intakes should be avoided in the LBW infant. Since the chloride content of breast milk is 11–22 mmol/l (1.6–3.3 mmol/100 kcal), the amount of chloride provided by most formulas (11–16 mmol/l (1.6–2.5 mmol/100 kcal)) would appear to be adequate to avoid chloride deficiency. At an energy intake of 130 kcal/kg/d they would provide 2.1–3.3 mmol/kg/d. At standard energy intake, both foods would provide 2.2–4.3 mmol/kg/d.

Iron. At 1 kg the fetus has 64 mg of iron, thereafter gaining 1.8 mg/kg/d. The iron stores of infants weighing less than 1.4 kg would be exhausted after 6–8 weeks, whereas those in heavier LBW infants would probably last to about 12 weeks postnatal age. Frequent blood sampling may deplete the infant's iron stores (1 g of haemoglobin contains 3 mg of iron) (5), although these infants appear to be able to compensate for such blood loss remarkably well (53).

As noted in chapter 2, iron-deficiency anaemia is extremely rare in normal infants fed only on breast milk during the first 6–8 months of life. There is, however, a physiological fall in haemoglobin concentration in the first two months of life and a redistribution of this iron to storage compartments (20). Preterm infants experience a fall in haemoglobin concentration during this same period that is more marked than in term infants. It seems that the fall varies with the birth weight, even if supposedly adequate iron supplementation is provided. Thus the so-called early anaemia of prematurity, which results in low haemoglobin values at two months of age, cannot be prevented by iron supplementation and should therefore be considered as physiological (20).

The absorption of iron from any milk is higher

in preterm than in full-term infants (54). Even VLBW infants (body weight < 1250 g) are apparently able to absorb the iron needed for their high requirements given their remarkably rapid rate of postnatal growth (20). It has been observed that exclusively human-milk-fed VLBW infants who were getting iron supplements from two months of age had a higher concentration of haemoglobin and serum ferritin at four months of age than another group that was formula fed and given supplementary iron from birth. This indicates that the small LBW infant absorbs supplementary iron better when fed on human milk than on formula (20).

Some studies appear to show that the premature infant cannot maintain optimal iron nutrition, without supplementation, after the age of two months (20). It is difficult to indicate what is the optimal dose of iron as supplement because individual needs for iron may vary with birth weight, neonatal sickness, and blood loss. Some data indicate that infants, whose birth weight ranged between 1 and 2 kg, who were given 2 mg of iron/kg/d, did not show clinical iron deficiency (55). The dose was probably adequate and was certainly not excessive for the maintenance of iron stores. However, many borderline serum ferritin values were found although no anaemia was documented (55). It could be argued that a higher dose of iron such as 3 mg/kg/d would provide a more comfortable margin of safety, especially in those infants with a birth weight between 1 and 1.5 kg. Some data indicate that 4 mg of iron/kg/d administered to a group of VLBW infants (birth weight < 1 kg) would prevent most laboratory signs of iron deficiency (53). There was, however, a marked decline in serum ferritin despite the large dose of iron administered.

Some proprietary formulas contain sufficient iron to achieve the recommended intake without any supplement. It is possible that excessive iron supplements are associated with an increased risk of lipid peroxidation and haemolytic anaemia, altered intestinal flora, and an increased risk of Gram-negative septicaemia. However, these risks have not been totally substantiated.

To achieve iron intakes of 2.0–2.5 mg/kg/d, infant formula should contain about 1.5 mg of iron per 100 kcal which, on the recommended range of energy intake, would supply 1.7–2.5 mg/kg/d at a formula content of 1–1.28 mg/dl. However, most formulas contain 0.6–0.7 mg of iron per dl, and infants fed on them may thus need supplementation at about 8 weeks of age. The maximum iron supplement should be 15 mg/d.

Since blood transfusions provide significant amounts of iron, infants who are having their haemoglobin concentrations maintained this way have no further need for iron supplements.

Copper (4, 56). The fetus accumulates copper at the rate of 51 μg/kg/d; at term, the infant has 14 mg of the element, half of which has accumulated in the liver during the last trimester of pregnancy. Sporadic copper deficiency occurs in LBW infants and its grossest manifestations are iron-resistant anaemia and skeletal changes. The copper requirements of the preterm infant have not been established and there appears to be no need for routine supplementation of breast-fed infants. An adequate copper content for proprietary formulas would be 90–120 μg/100 kcal, which would provide between 120–150 μg/kg/d.

Zinc (4, 5). The fetus' zinc content is fairly constant at 19 ± 5 mg/kg fat-free tissue. During the last trimester the accumulation of zinc is 149 μg/kg/d; thus a full-term infant has about 66 mg of the element, 25% of which is in the liver and 40% in the skeleton. Although there is no specific systemic store of zinc in the term or preterm infant, redistribution of this hepatic and skeletal zinc may be able to meet the demands of newly synthesized lean tissue. However, symptomatic zinc deficiency occasionally occurs in LBW infants at 2.5–4.5 months postnatal age. It is not known whether these infants develop zinc deficiency because of the low zinc content of breast milk or because of their high rates of growth relative to zinc supply. Both factors are probably important.

The characteristic features of zinc deficiency (dermatitis, poor feeding, slowed weight gain, frequent loose stools, irritability, jitteriness and, sometimes, convulsions) disappear rapidly with oral zinc supplements (15–61 μmol/kg/d). It has been suggested that proprietary formulas for preterm infants should contain 0.55–1.1 mg/100 kcal (0.72–1.44 mg/kg/d at an intake of 130 kcal/kg/d).

Fat-soluble vitamins

Vitamin A (3, 5). The molar ratio of retinal:retinol-binding protein is lower in LBW preterm infants than in infants born at term. Although overt vitamin A deficiency in the former is rare, low plasma retinol levels may be associated with functional biochemical evidence of deficiency. This suggests a need to supply additional vitamin A, which is further strengthened by the likelihood of increased requirements arising from the deposition of the vitamin in adipose tissue. Vitamin A utilization increases in infants who are being ventilated, and this has been associated with the development of bronchopulmonary dysplasia (57), although there is as yet no clear evidence that this is a causal association.

It has been suggested that preterm infants

should receive between 200 and 1000 μg of vitamin A daily. Breast milk contains about 90 μg of vitamin A per 100 kcal and it has been proposed that the content of proprietary formulas for LBW infants should be not less than this, with an upper limit of 150 μg/100 kcal. The intake at which vitamin A toxicity develops is unclear. Certainly many infants receive much larger doses of vitamin A adventitiously with the use of multivitamin supplements to achieve adequate vitamin D intakes.

Vitamin D (5, 58). The amount of vitamin D in the fetus is dependent upon the mother's intake and exposure to sunlight. Congenital neonatal rickets has been described in LBW infants born to vitamin D-deficient mothers; otherwise overt vitamin D deficiency is of later onset. Since the intestinal mucosa responds poorly to 1-25-dihydroxy-cholecalciferol before 32 weeks gestation, and because of difficulties in optimizing calcium and phosphorus metabolism, LBW infants may need vitamin D supplements. If they are breast-fed, a suitable dose would be 1000 IU (25 μg/d), with a range of 800–1600 IU/d. There is a risk of hypercalcaemia if infant formula is supplemented with vitamin D; it is preferable if such products do not contain more than 120 IU (3 μg)/100 kcal, as cholecalciferol or ergocalciferol. Supplements can then be more easily regulated and provided in similar doses to those for breast-fed infants.

Vitamin E (3, 5). Vitamin E activity comprises 8 different compounds, all of which are lipid-soluble, membrane-related, free-radical scavengers or antioxidants. The requirement for vitamin E has not been established. It varies with oxidative stress, which in turn is related to iron intake and to the susceptibility of tissue membranes to oxidative damage; thus infants on high intakes of polyunsaturated fatty acids (PUFA) have increased vitamin-E requirements, which are expressed frequently in relation to PUFA intake.

The possibility that pharmacological doses of vitamin E may prevent bronchopulmonary dysplasia, retinopathy of the preterm and intraventricular haemorrhage has not been fully substantiated and should not, as yet, serve as a basis for recommended vitamin-E intakes. Breast milk, which contains 0.29–0.54 mg tocopherol equivalents (TE) per dl, has a TE:PUFA ratio of 0.7–1.1 mg/g. This exceeds that which has been found to prevent lipid peroxidation and symptomatic vitamin E deficiency (as manifested by erythrocytic sensitivity to peroxide haemolysis and altered platelet function). As an extension of these observations, it has been proposed that the vitamin-E content of proprietary formulas should not be below 0.4 mg TE/dl (0.6 mg/100 kcal) at a ratio of alpha-tocopherol:PUFA of 0.9 mg/g.

Vitamin K (5). Vitamin K is required for a number of carboxylation mechanisms, which involve the formation of carboxyglutamate. This is found in the coagulation factors prothrombin, VII, IX and X; osteocalcin, which is a possible site of interaction with vitamin D; and in a renal tubular protein, which may solubilize urinary calcium.

LBW infants need vitamin K supplements because of their rapid systemic utilization of this vitamin, low dietary intake, and limited intestinal production possibilities. Standard practice is to give all infants 0.5–1 mg of vitamin K intramuscularly on the first day of life. This can be repeated at weekly intervals until the child is on adequate oral feeding, which should provide 2–3 μg/kg/d. Most proprietary formulas contain 3–10 μg vitamin K per dl and the amount in breast milk is slightly lower at 1–2 μg/dl.

Water-soluble vitamins

Thiamin (5). Thiamin deficiency (beriberi) is rare in LBW infants unless they have been breast-fed by thiamin-deficient mothers or fed soy-based formula. Normally there is sufficient thiamin in breast milk to maintain an adequate supply for infants. However, since this vitamin is inactivated by heat treatment, the thiamin content of pasteurized breast milk is low, and supplements may be needed to ensure an intake of 25 μg/kg/d. It has been suggested that proprietary formulas should contain sufficient thiamin to provide an intake of 20 μg/100 kcal (15 μg/dl). Intakes of 10 times this amount have been tolerated by LBW infants.

Riboflavin (5, 59). The case for ensuring a minimum intake of riboflavin in preterm infants is based on demonstration of biochemical riboflavin deficiency and on evidence that riboflavin may increase the efficacy of phototherapy. Intakes of 40–60 μg/100 kcal are probably adequate. Breast milk contains 30–50 μg/dl (40–70 μg/100 kcal), while most proprietary formulas have a higher content still. Since riboflavin is photosensitive, it has been argued that the exposure of breast milk to light results in a variable loss of vitamin activity. In addition, phototherapy may cause a transient biochemical riboflavin deficiency in breast-fed infants, although no clinical signs of such deficiencies have been reported.

Nicotinic acid (niacin) (5). This vitamin is synthesized endogenously from tryptophan; 60 mg of tryptophan yields 1 mg of niacin and is defined as one niacin equivalent (NE). Total NE in dietary intakes is equivalent to niacin (mg) plus (0.017 × tryptophan (mg)). Since neither pellagra nor nicotinic-acid toxicity has been observed in LBW infants, there is probably no need to supplement the intake of breast-fed infants. Breast milk contains 0.6 NE/dl (0.85 NE/100 kcal); it has therefore been suggested that proprietary formulas should contain 0.5–1.0 mg niacin per dl, in addition to their variable tryptophan content, to achieve a minimum intake of 0.8 NE/100 kcal.

Pyridoxine (vitamin B₆) (5). Pyridoxine, pyridoxal and pyridoxamine have similar activities. Deficiencies in LBW infants are manifested by vomiting, irritability, dermatitis, failure to thrive and convulsions. The possibility of such a deficiency increases with the use of such drugs as isoniazid and penicillamine. Pyridoxine intake may best be assessed relative to protein intake. Breast milk contains 35 µg of pyridoxine per 100 kcal, which is approximately 15 µg/g protein, and it has been suggested that proprietary formulas should contain similar amounts. No upper limit has been established and toxicity has not been observed at intakes as high as 250 µg/100 kcal.

Pantothenic acid (5). Neither clinical deficiency nor toxicity of this vitamin has been observed in the LBW infant. It has therefore been suggested that proprietary formulas should contain about 200 µg/dl (330 µg/100 kcal), which matches the content of breast milk (200–400 µg/dl).

Biotin (5). Biotin, which is readily absorbed, is produced by intestinal microflora. With the exception of infants on total parenteral nutrition, no deficiency has been observed. Since breast milk contains 0.8 µg biotin per dl, proprietary formulas should probably match this (about 1 µg/dl (1.5 µg/100 kcal)).

Folic acid (5). Deficiency of folic acid in LBW infants has a profound effect on cell division, leading to megaloblastic anaemia, leucopenia, thrombocytopenia, impaired growth, intestinal villous atrophy and altered maturation of the CNS. Folate deficiency in LBW infants has been readily corrected by daily supplements of 60–65 µg of folic acid; nevertheless, the criteria for adequate folate supply are not clear. The content of breast milk varies but normally provides 65 µg daily. Most standard proprietary formulas contain at least 40 µg of folic acid per dl (approximately 60 µg/100 kcal). Since folic acid is heat-sensitive, the possibility of a folate deficiency developing in infants who are fed heat-treated formulas should not be overlooked.

Vitamin B₁₂ (6). Proprietary formulas contain more vitamin B₁₂ (0.1–2 µg/dl) than does breast milk (0.1 µg/dl). However, clinical B₁₂ deficiency has not been seen in LBW infants unless they have been breast-fed by vitamin B₁₂-deficient mothers or by strict vegans. There is, therefore, no need to supplement the intakes of either breast-fed or proprietary formula-fed infants.

Ascorbic acid (vitamin C) (3, 5). Vitamin C is essential for the conversion of folic acid to folinic acid, and the hydroxylation of proline, lysine, adrenalin and tryptophan. It is a powerful reducing agent and a consequent adventitious effect may be that, at adequate dosage, it prevents the transient hypertyrosinaemia and hyperphenylalaninaemia seen in LBW infants, especially those who are on high-protein intakes. Vitamin C may present the additional advantage of being a systemic antioxidant.

Breast milk contains about 4 mg vitamin C per dl, although this can be reduced by as much as 90% through heat treatment. Proprietary formulas supply 5–30 mg/dl. The ideal intake of vitamin C has not been established but it is clearly prudent to ensure adequate intake. Consequently, it has been recommended that breast-fed infants receive at least 20 mg of vitamin C daily and that proprietary formulas contain at least 5 mg of vitamin C per dl (7.5 mg/100 kcal). These intakes may have to be increased in infants fed on casein-dominant formulas.

Résumé

Le nourrisson de petit poids de naissance

Environ 16% des enfants qui naissent dans le monde pèsent moins de 2500 g. En dessous de cette limite on distingue ceux qui pèsent entre 1,5 et 1 kg et ceux qui pèsent moins de 1 kg. Ces nouveaux-nés ont des besoins nutritionnels particuliers du fait de leur croissance extrêmement rapide et de leur immaturité. La prise en charge nutritionnelle des nourrissons de faible poids de naissance a fait l'objet d'études très complètes et des recommandations ont été formulées. Le rapport de la Société européenne de gastro-entérologie pédiatrique et de nutrition (SEGEPN) sur "L'alimentation et la nutrition des prématurés" fait aussi le point sur la question.

Il n'y a pas de critères idéaux pour la prise en charge nutritionnelle des enfants de poids insuffisant à la naissance. On ne peut se baser sur les critères de croissance intra-utérine pour fixer les critères postnatals, d'abord parce que les besoins métaboliques diffèrent, ensuite parce que les prématurés perdent très vite des liquides extracellulaires pour arriver à un rapport liquides extracellulaires-liquides intracellulaires équivalant à celui des enfants nés à terme, ce qui représente une perte de poids de 8 à 10%. Les apports conseillés qui sont donnés ici ne représentent pas des besoins physiologiques vérifiés.

De manière générale les enfants nés après 35 semaines de gestation ou plus, et qui constituent la grande majorité des prématurés, peuvent et devraient recevoir du lait maternel. S'il peut être nécessaire d'enrichir le lait de la mère pour les quelques enfants nés entre la 32ème et la 35ème semaine de gestation, virtuellement tous peuvent être nourris au sein ou au moins avec du lait maternel. Les prématurés nés avant la 32ème semaine, dont la plupart ont un poids de naissance inférieur à 1500 g, représentent un groupe particulier du fait de leurs besoins nutritionnels particulièrement élevés. Au début une alimentation parentérale pourra être nécessaire.

Techniques d'alimentation

Les techniques choisies doivent compenser l'immaturité de l'enfant et ne pas risquer de perturber la circulation de l'air ou de favoriser une aspiration du contenu de l'estomac. Durant la période initiale pour les nourrissons de très faible poids de naissance ou d'extrêmement faible poids de naissance ni la voie orale directe ni le sondage ne sont possibles. C'est donc une alimentation parentérale totale qui est nécessaire. Ceci est valable aussi pour les enfants malades. Bien que la déglutition apparaisse dès la 16ème semaine, une activité motrice organisée de l'œsophage ne se développe pas avant environ la 34ème semaine ce qui explique la prédisposition des prématurés au reflux œsophagien. Des apports massifs sont mal tolérés, la capacité gastrique limitée peut gêner les fonctions respiratoires en cas de distension. Il faudra souvent combiner alimentation parentérale et alimentation par la voie digestive.

La vidange gastrique est plus rapide avec le lait de femme qu'avec d'autres formules et elle est favorisée en procubitus et en position latérale. Il est recommandé d'utiliser des sondes en silicone plutôt qu'en PVC afin de diminuer le risque de perforation intestinale. Les avantages d'un sondage transpylorique par rapport à un sondage intragastrique sont discutés. La sonde transpylorique ne prédispose probablement pas au risque d'entérocolite nécrosante et la localisation de la sonde dans le duodénum plutôt que dans le jéjunum évite des problèmes d'absorption, notamment des lipides. Le fait d'utiliser une infusion entérale continue ou intermittente demeure sujet à controverse.

Ce chapitre examine successivement les différents besoins.

Eau. Les pertes en eau qui conditionnent les besoins peuvent être réduites, pour les pertes extra rénales, par le maintien des prématurés en atmosphère humidifiée à 80% ou plus. Le volume urinaire dépend quant à lui de la charge osmotique imposée au rein. Même si le système arginine-vasopressine est stimulé au maximum ces nouveau-nés ne peuvent atteindre une osmolalité supérieure à 500 mOsm/kg. En fonction des pertes les besoins quotidiens en eau sont donc de 150 à 200 ml/kg de poids corporel.

Energie. Au repos le métabolisme est plus élevé que chez les enfants à terme, il est de 36 à 60 kcal/kg/j. En tenant compte de tous les autres facteurs on pense que les besoins sont satisfaits avec un apport journalier calorique de 120 à 130 kcal/kg.

Protéines. Les besoins ont été estimés à 2,9 et 3,5 g/kg/j à 24 et 36 semaines respectivement. La taurine pourrait intervenir dans la croissance mais il n'est pas certain qu'il faille systématiquement en enrichir le régime, même si l'on pense que les formules spéciales doivent être enrichies en taurine pour atteindre la même concentration que dans le lait maternel. Les protéines doivent en règle générale représenter environ 10% de la ration.

Lipides. 50% de l'énergie fournie par le lait maternel l'est sous forme de lipides et ceci aussi bien chez les mères ayant accouché prématurément que chez celles ayant accouché à terme. La SEGEPN recommande que les formules spéciales pour prématurés ne contiennent pas plus de 40% de triglycérides à chaînes moyennes. Quantitativement pour un apport énergétique de 130 kcal/kg/j, avec des apports en glucides et en protéines maximum, les apports conseillés seraient de 4,7 g/kg (soit 3,6 g/100 kcal). Les apports pourraient aller de 4 à 9 g/kg/j avec une densité lipidique maximum de 7 g/100 kcal dans les préparations. Comme pour la taurine il a été suggéré d'enrichir les régimes avec de la carnitine de manière à fournir 60 à 90 μmol/l, le lait maternel contenant 39 à 63 μmol/l.

Glucides. Le lait maternel contient 7 à 8 g de lactose/dl (7,7 g/100 kcal) et ne doit donc pas être enrichi. On propose pour les formules spéciales une teneur en lactose de 3,2 à 12 g/100 kcal ne dépassant pas 8 g/dl. Ainsi la teneur totale recommandée de la ration en glucides est de 7 à 14 g/100 kcal avec un maximum de 11 g/dl. Des apports supérieurs pourraient être envisagés mais ils risqueraient de provoquer une diarrhée osmotique et un déséquilibre du rapport énergie/protéines.

Minéraux. (Les chiffres donnés se rapportent à la teneur en sels minéraux des formules ou préparations spéciales pour prématurés)

— Calcium et phosphate: La SEGEPN recommande pour le calcium un apport de 1,75 à 3,5 mmol/100 kcal et pour le phosphore un apport de 1,6 à 2,9 mmol/100 kcal.
— Magnésium: 6 à 12 mg/100 kcal (0,25 à 0,5 mmol/100 kcal).
— Sodium: 6,5 à 15 mmol Na/l (1,0 à 2,3 mmol/100 kcal).
— Potassium: 15 à 25 mmol/l.
— Chlorures: 11 à 16 mmol/l (1,6 à 2,5 mmol/100 kcal).
— Fer: 1,5 mg/100 kcal.
— Cuivre: 90 à 100 μg/100 kcal soit 120 à 150 μg/kg/j.
— Zinc: 0,55 à 1,1 mg/100 kcal.

Vitamines liposolubles

— Vitamine A: Les prématurés doivent recevoir 200 à 1000 μg/j avec une limite de 150 μg/100 kcal dans les formules spéciales.
— Vitamine D: 800 à 1600 UI/j.
— Vitamine E: Les formules spéciales devraient contenir au moins 0,4 ET/dl (0,6 mg/100 kcal) (ET = équivalent tocophérol).
— Vitamine K: 0,5 à 1 mg intramusculaire le premier jour de la vie.

Vitamines hydrosolubles

— Thiamine: L'apport doit être de 25 μg/kg/j.
— Riboflavine: L'apport doit être de 40 à 60 μg/100 kcal.
— Acide nicotinique (B3): Les formules doivent contenir 0,5 à 1 mg (dl de niacine).
— Pyridoxine (B_6): Il n'y a pas de toxicité même avec des apports de l'ordre de 250 μg/100 kcal.
— Acide pantothénique: 200 μg/dl (330 μg/100 kcal) dans les formules.
— Biotine. 1 μg/dl (1,5 μg/100 kcal dans les formules.
— Acide folique: 40 μg/dl (60 μg/100 kcal) dans les formules.
— Vitamine B_{12}: Il n'est pas nécessaire d'enrichir le régime.

— Acide ascorbique (vitamine C): 5 mg/dl (7,5 mg/100 kcal) dans les formules.

En conclusion le choix entre le lait maternel et les formules de substitution dans l'alimentation des nourrissons de poids insuffisant à la naissance est très difficile aussi bien du point de vue des justifications nutritionnelles et immunologiques que d'un point de vue pratique. Etant donné que la plupart (>90%) de ces nourrissons naissent dans les pays en développement l'utilisation du lait de la mère pourrait être la seule option réaliste. Toutefois, indépendamment de la nature des systèmes de santé, des niveaux technologiques ou des formules alternatives disponibles, des études ont démontré qu'il y a avantage à alimenter les nourrissons de poids insuffisant à la naissance avec le lait de leur propre mère quel que soit l'environnement.

References

1. **Milner, R.D.G.** Metabolic and endocrine responses in weight: an update. *Wkly epidemiol. rec.,* **59**(27): 205–211 (1984).
2. **Kramer, M.S.** Determinants of low birth weight: methodological assessment and meta-analysis. *Bull. Wld Hlth Org.,* **65**: 663–737 (1987).
3. **Brooke, O.G.** Nutritional requirements of low and very low-birth-weight infants. *Ann. rev. nutr.,* **7**: 91–116 (1987).
4. **Shaw, J.C.L.** Growth and nutrition of the very preterm infant. *Br. med. bull.,* **44**: 984–1009 (1988).
5. **Committee on the Nutrition of the Preterm Infant. European Society of Paediatric Gastroenterology and Nutrition.** *Nutrition and feeding of preterm infants.* Oxford, Blackwell Scientific Publications, 1987.
6. **Canadian Pediatric Society. Committee on Nutrition.** Feeding the low-birth-weight infant. *Can. Med. Assoc. j.,* **124**: 1301–1311 (1981).
7. **American Academy of Pediatrics: Committee on Nutrition.** Nutritional needs of low-birth-weight infants. *Pediatrics,* **75**: 976–986 (1985).
8. **Milner, R.D.G.** Metabolic and endocrine responses in enteral and parenteral feeding of the preterm infant. In: Taylor, T.G. & Jenkins, N.K., ed. *Proceedings of the XIII International Congress of Nutrition.* London, John Libbey, 1986, pp. 636–639.
9. **Milla, P.J. & Bisset, W.M.** The gastrointestinal tract. *Br. med. bull.,* **44**: 1010–1024 (1988).
10. **Raiha, N.C.R.** Handicaps of amino acid metabolism and optimal protein nutrition of preterm infants. In: Freier, S. & Eidelman, A.I., ed. *Human milk: its biological and social value.* Amsterdam, Excerpta Medica, 1980, pp. 15–22.
11. **Pearce, J.L. & Buchanan, L.F.** Breast milk and breast-feeding in very low-birth-weight infants. *Arch. dis. child.,* **54**: 897–899 (1979).

12. **Smallpeice, V. & Davies, P.A.** Immediate feeding of premature infants with undiluted breast milk. *Lancet*, **2**: 1349–1352 (1964).
13. **Davies, P.A. & Russel, H.** Later progress of 100 infants weighing 1000 to 2000 g at birth fed immediately with breast milk. *Devel. med. child neurol.*, **10**: 725–735 (1968).
14. **Fanaroff, A.A. & Klaus, M.H.** The gastrointestinal tract—feeding and selected disorders. In: Klaus, M.H. & Fanaroff, A.A., ed. *Care of the high-risk neonate*, 2nd ed. Philadelphia, Saunders, 1979.
15. **Morley, R. et al.** Mother's choice to provide breast milk and developmental outcome. *Arch. dis. child.*, **63**: 1382–1385 (1988).
16. **Heird, W.C.** Advances in infant nutrition over the past quarter century. *J. Am. Coll. Nutr. (special issue)*, **8(S)**: 22S–32S (1989).
17. **Gross, S.J. et al.** Nutritional composition of milk produced by mothers delivering preterm. *J. pediatr.*, **77**: 641–644 (1980).
18. **Lemons, J.A. et al.** Differences in the composition of preterm and term milk during early lactation. *Pediatr. res.*, **16**: 113–117 (1982).
19. Breast not necessarily best. *Lancet*, **1**: 624–626 (1988) (Editorial).
20. **Siimes, M.A.** Iron nutrition in low-birth-weight infants. In: Stekel. A., ed. *Iron nutrition in infancy and childhood*. Nestlé Nutrition Workshop Series, Vol. 4. New York, Raven Press, 1984, pp. 75–94.
21. **Rönnholm, K.A.R. et al.** Human milk protein supplementation for the prevention of hypoproteinemia without metabolic imbalance in breast-milk-fed very-low-birth-weight infants. *J. pediatr.*, **101**: 243–247 (1982).
22. **Rönnholm, K.A.R. et al.** Supplementation with human milk protein improves growth of small premature infants fed human milk. *Pediatrics*, **77**: 649–653 (1986).
23. **Campbell, N.** Breast milk feeding of sick babies. *Breastfeeding rev.*, **6**: 8–12 (1985).
24. **Singhania, A.B. & Sharma, J.N.** Fortified high-calorie human milk for optimal growth of low-birth-weight babies. *J. trop. pediatr.*, **35**: 77–81 (1989).
25. **Singh, M.** *Care of the newborn.* New Delhi, Sagar Publications, 1985, p. 124.
26. **Bagui, B.N. & Daga, A.S.** Reduction in neonatal mortality with simple interventions. *J. trop. ped.*, **35**: 191–196 (1989).
27. **Armstrong, H.C.** Breastfeeding low birthweight babies: advances in Kenya. *J. of hum. lac.*, **3**: 34–37 (1987).
28. **Meier, P.** Bottle- and breast-feeding: effects on transcutaneous oxygen pressure and temperature in preterm infants. *Nurs. res.*, **37**: 36–41 (1988).
29. **Steichen, J. et al.** Breast-feeding the low-birth-weight preterm infant. *Clinics in perinatology*, **14**: 131–172 (1987).
30. **Schnaler, R.J. et al.** Fortified mother's milk for very low-birth-weight infants: results of growth and nutrient balance studies. *J. pediatr.*, **107**: 437–445 (1987).
31. **Rutter, N.** The immature skin. *Br. med. bull.*, **44**: 957–970 (1988).
32. **Hammarlund, R. & Sedin, G.** Transepidermal water loss in newborn infants. III. Relation to gestational age. *Acta pediatr. scand.*, **68**: 795–801 (1979).
33. **Coulthard, M. & Hey, E.N.** Effect of varying water intake on renal functions in healthy preterm babies. *Arch. dis. child.*, **60**: 614–620 (1985).
34. **Rees, L. et al.** Hyponatraemia in the first week of life in preterm infants. I. Arginine-vasopressin secretion. *Arch. dis. child.*, **59**: 414–422 (1984).
35. **Sinclair, J.C.** ed. *Temperature regulation and energy metabolism in the newborn.* New York, Grune & Stratton, 1978.
36. **Reichman, B.L. et al.** Partition of energy metabolism and energy cost of growth in the very low-birth-weight infant. *Pediatrics*, **69**: 446–451 (1982).
37. **Chessex, P. et al.** Metabolic consequences of intrauterine growth retardation in very low-birth-weight infants. *Pediatr. res.*, **18**: 709–713 (1984).
38. **Jackson, A.A. et al.** Nitrogen metabolism in preterm infants fed human donor breast milk: the possible essentiality of glycine. *Pediatr. res.*, **15**: 1454–1461 (1981).
39. **Kashyap, S. et al.** Growth, nutrient retention, and metabolic response in low-birth-weight infants fed varying intakes of protein and energy. *J. pediatr.*, **113**: 713–721 (1988).
40. **Rönholm, K.A.R. et al.** Supplementation with human-milk protein improves growth of small premature infants fed human milk. *Pediatrics*, **77**: 649–653 (1986).
41. **Putet, G. et al.** Supplementation of pooled human milk with casein hydrolysate: energy and nitrogen balance and weight gain composition in very low-birth-weight infants. *Ped. res.*, **21**: 458–461 (1987).
42. **Chesney, R.W.** Taurine: is it required for infant nutrition? *J. nutr.*, **118**: 6–10 (1988).
43. **Clandinin, M.T. et al.** Do low-birth-weight infants require nutrition with chain elongation desaturation products of essential fatty acids? *Prog. lipid res.*, **10**: 901–904 (1982).
44. **Lucas, A.** Does diet in preterm infants influence clinical outcome? *Biology of the neonate*, **52** (suppl. 1): 141–146 (1987).
45. **Kalhan, S.C. et al.** Estimation of glucose turnover and 13C recycling in the human newborn by simultaneous [1-13C] glucose and [6,6-1H2] glucose tracers. *J. clin. endocrinol. metab.*, **50**: 456–460 (1980).
46. **Lucas, A. et al.** Adverse neurodevelopmental outcome of moderate neonatal hypoglycaemia. *Br. med. j.*, **297**: 1304–1308 (1988).
47. **Filer, L.J., ed.** Assessment of bone mineralization in infants. *J. pediatr.*, **113**: 165–248 (1988).
48. **McIntosh, N. et al.** Plasma 25-hydroxyvitamin D and rickets in low-birth-weight infants. *Arch. dis. child.*, **58**: 476–477 (1983).
49. **Gross, S.J.** Bone mineralization in preterm infants fed human milk with and without mineral supplementation. *J. pediatr.*, **111**: 450–458 (1987).
50. **Brooke, O.G. & Lucas, A.** Metabolic bone disease in

preterm infants. *Arch. dis. child.*, **60**: 682−685 (1985).

51. **Senterre, J. et al.** Effects of vitamin D and phosphorus supplementation on calcium retention in preterm infants fed banked human milk. *J. pediatr.*, **103**: 305−307 (1983).

52. **Carey, D.E. et al.** Phosphorus wasting during phosphorus supplementation of human milk feedings in preterm infants. *J. pediatr.*, **107**: 790−794 (1985).

53. **Siimes, M.A. & Järvenpää, A.L.** Prevention of anaemia and iron deficiency in very low-birth-weight infants. *J. pediatr.*, **101**: 277−280 (1982).

54. **Dauncy, M.J. et al.** The effect of iron supplements and blood transfusion on iron absorption by low-birth-weight infants fed pasteurized human breast milk. *Pediatr. res.*, **12**: 899−904 (1978).

55. **Lundström, U. et al.** At what age does iron supplementation become necessary in low-birth-weight infants? *J. pediatr.*, **91**: 878–883 (1977).

56. Copper and the infant. *Lancet*, **1**: 900−901 (1987) (Editorial).

57. **Shenai, J.P. et al.** Vitamin A status of neonates with chronic lung disease. *Pediatr. res.*, **19**: 185−189 (1985).

58. **Tsang, R.C.** The quandary of vitamin D in the newborn infant. *Lancet*, **1**: 1370−1372 (1983).

59. **Lucas, A. & Bates, C.** Transient riboflavin depletion in preterm infants. *Arch. dis. child.*, **59**: 837−841 (1984).

6. The infant and young child during periods of acute infection

Passive immunity, which is conferred on infants through maternal antibodies and breast milk, helps to protect them against infection during the first months of life. Later, as this immunity decreases and contact with the environment increases, the incidence of infections rises rapidly and persists at a high level during the second and third years of life. Infections and inadequate diet may be of little consequence for the well-nourished child; in underweight children, however, each episode of infection is frequently more protracted and has a considerably greater impact on health. Besides the reduced food intake and absorption, the demand for nutrients is higher during periods of infectious diseases. Infants who are exclusively breast-fed are at much lower risk from diarrhoeal diseases. In contrast, bottle-fed infants and children receiving foods other than milk, particularly in an unsanitary environment, are at much greater risk of infection from contaminated food and utensils. The period of convalescence from diarrhoeal and other disease is characterized by the return of a normal appetite and increased nutritional requirements to permit catch-up growth and the replenishment of nutritional reserves. A primary requirement is that children receive sufficient dietary energy and nutrients to enable them to achieve their growth potential.

Introduction

During the first months of life, infants are relatively well protected against most diseases through passive immunity from maternal antibodies transmitted through the placenta and persisting in the blood for the first 3–4 months of life. Protection is stronger and lasts longer if infants are breast-fed. As discussed in chapter 2, breast-feeding protects infants against most common infectious diseases through a number of very efficient mechanisms (1, 2).

During the second half of the breast-fed infant's first year of life, the proportion of breast milk gradually decreases in the overall diet while at the same time the child's contact with the environment increases. As a consequence, the incidence of infections, particularly diarrhoeal diseases, rises rapidly and persists at a high level during the second and third years of life (3, 4). In situations where living conditions are characterized by poor environmental sanitation and overcrowding, acute infectious diseases constitute the major cause of morbidity and mortality in children (5). The incidence of infections usually decreases after the third year as children's resistance to disease builds up.

The situation is similar for children who are not breast-fed. However, the incidence of diarrhoeal diseases is higher and begins earlier, both because of the absence of the protection that breast milk affords and because of the greater risk of infections associated with bottle-feeding (6).

Overall, it is difficult to determine whether the main cause of growth retardation is infectious diseases or inadequate diet. What is clear, however, is that the two act synergistically, each aggravating the effects of the other (7). The combined impact of infectious diseases and inadequate diet during illness may be of little consequence for well-nourished children for whom such incidents are, for the most part, infrequent, self-limiting and short in duration. Furthermore, these children have an opportunity to recover fully after each episode, and they generally receive a healthy diet during convalescence. In underweight children, however, episodes of infection are frequently more protracted.

Studies in the Gambia (8) and in Sudan (9) show very little impact of diarrhoea on growth among exclusively breast-fed infants. The situation can be radically different, however, for children whose normal dietary intake is marginally adequate, or even frankly insufficient. This is the case during the weaning period for many children in developing countries who are fed high-fibre, high-bulk foods of low nutritional value at the same time as they are suffering from infectious diseases. Frequent infections are largely responsible for the high mortality rates among infants and young children in these countries and for the retardation in growth and development of many of the survivors.

Effects of infections on nutritional status

The mechanisms by which infections can be harmful to the nutritional status of children include (10):

— reduced food and water intake due to anorexia and/or other reasons for withholding food;
— diminished absorption and utilization of ingested food;
— increased nutrient and water losses;

— increased metabolic demands and therefore higher nutritional requirements;
— alteration of metabolic pathways;
— intentional reduction, or complete withholding, of food.

Anorexia and other conditions

It is a common clinical observation that children on their own eat less when suffering from infectious diseases. Experimental studies have been carried out in animals (11, 12) to try to understand the mechanisms that are responsible for the accompanying reduction in appetite. For example, fever and a significantly reduced food intake resulted when animals were injected with an endotoxin. Even when the fever was controlled by administering antipyretic drugs, food intake was still lower than among controls. In cases where tolerance to the endotoxin had been conferred by previous injections, the animals had an attenuated reaction when injected again, including a lower rise in temperature, and their food intake was no different from that of the controls. These studies suggest that, far from being caused by the presence of fever, anorexia is part of the mechanism by which an organism reacts to infection.

Other studies suggest that anorexia is mediated by interleukin-1, which is released by infected macrophages. Many metabolic effects of interleukin-1 have been reviewed (13), and a particularly interesting action is the release of lactoferrin from neutrophil-specific granules. The lactoferrin binds iron, thus causing a reduction in plasma iron. Similarly, interleukin-1 stimulates the synthesis of metallothionine causing a reduction of plasma zinc, and caeruloplasmin production, which is reflected in the increase of bound serum copper during infection.

It is well recognized that microbial growth is stimulated by the presence of zinc and iron. Perhaps the reduction of plasma zinc and iron are a protective mechanism during the early stages of infection. An explanation of the pathophysiology of kwashiorkor in terms of the action of free radicals has been put forward (14). The body's defence is to produce free radicals in sufficient quantity to kill invading organisms. Free radicals are chemical compounds, for example superoxide and hydrogen peroxide, that are capable of damaging tissues through their action on lipid membranes. Toxins and stimulated leukocytes produce large quantities of free radicals. A major catalyst of reactions with free radicals is iron which changes between the ferrous and ferric forms through redox cycling. The presence of abundant storage iron thus enhances the damaging effects of free radicals.

Iron deficiency is associated with impaired cellular immunity and bactericidal activity, which may increase the prevalence of respiratory infection and diarrhoea (15) among subjects living in highly infected environments. However, if large doses of iron are administered to subjects, especially by injection in the leg, rates of infection may increase (16). The practice of "starving a fever" is common in many traditional societies, sometimes on the advice of a health worker. Although this has obvious nutritional implications, it is possible that this "cultural control strategy" happens to complement the biological "infection control strategy".

Even mild, non-febrile infections can result in anorexia. The overall effect on food intake can be significant if the infections are frequent or prolonged. In a study undertaken in an effort to quantify the reduction in food intake associated with infectious diseases in children (17), it was found that, on average, energy or protein intake was reduced by about 20%. The reduction was greater still in cases of diarrhoea. These results occurred despite efforts to ensure adequate food intake for all children through dietary supplementation and by providing nutrition education for mothers.

In another study performed at a rural hospital treatment centre in Bangladesh (18), it was found that children had a reduced food intake of about 40% during diarrhoea. Some of these children were breast-fed, and it is interesting to note that their breast-milk intake at least was not affected. The conclusion from these and several other studies is that the "traditional" practice of withholding food from sick children is less significant as a cause for decreased food intake during diarrhoea than children's refusal to feed because they are feeling ill. However, because both of these studies were based on field observations in which children continued to live in their homes, it is impossible to determine to what extent the reduction in food intake was due to anorexia or related to the intentional withholding of food by mothers.

In a more controlled study (19), hospitalized children suffering from short-term diarrhoea accompanied by mild-to-moderate dehydration were fed *ad libitum* after their dehydration was corrected. Food intake during the acute stage of diarrhoea was between 45% and 64% of estimated energy requirements, depending on the etiology of the diarrhoea, the reduction being greatest in cases of rotavirus infection. It thus appears that there is a genuine physiological basis for reduced food intake by children during periods of acute infectious diseases.

There may be additional reasons for poor dietary intake, for example vomiting, which is a frequently observed symptom in young children during the initial stages of acute infections. It is one of the main reasons why mothers are afraid to feed their children during periods of acute infection and may thus contribute to reduced food intake, although there are no controlled studies about its significance. Dehydration during severe diarrhoea may cause a very dry buccal mucosa. *Monilia* infection of the buccal mucosa is common among children with severe protein-energy malnutrition, and is especially frequent among children with measles. The resulting infection of the tongue and lip lesions may combine to reduce dietary intake since solid foods are less easily swallowed than liquids in such circumstances. An infection may have little nutritional impact for infants who receive most of their dietary energy in the form of breast milk. However, a considerable reduction in energy intake during infection may result in older children, who customarily receive more than half of their energy via solid foods.

Impaired nutrient absorption and nutrient loss

The physiology of intestinal absorption is relatively well understood and many mechanisms of nutrient malabsorption have been described. Destruction of villi, leading to a decrease in surface area and reduction in brush-border enzymes, is of considerable importance. In addition, deconjugation of bile salts and reduction of their concentration in luminal fluid can lead to steatorrhoea. The secretory response in the intestinal mucosa, which is stimulated by bacterial toxins, can also result in malabsorption.

Nutrient malabsorption is not normally of concern during a single acute infectious episode. It may become nutritionally significant, however, where conditions are prolonged or acute episodes are frequent. This is related to accelerated gastrointestinal transit, transitory enzymatic deficiencies and morphological changes of the intestinal mucosa that usually occur during diarrhoea. The malabsorption of fats, carbohydrates and proteins is well documented (20, 21). The absorption of certain vitamins (folate, B_{12} and vitamin A) and minerals (magnesium, zinc and possibly others) has also been shown to be reduced.

Malnutrition during malabsorption may develop as a result of poor food intake, impaired digestion, decreased nutrient absorption, exudative losses of endogenous nutrients and changes in intraluminal metabolism (22). A variety of metabolic responses occur during infection, and they have profound effects on the use of dietary intake and endogenous nutrient stores. There is an increase in energy expenditure, in the range of 10–15% per 1°C rise in body temperature. Although not without nutritional implications for an anorexic individual who is not being offered much food, fever has a number of immunological advantages. Most immune systems are more active at 39°C than at 37°C. The metabolic changes during infection are reviewed elsewhere; it is clear,

however, that carbohydrate stores for fuel are rapidly depleted, the effective use of fat is inhibited, and obligatory gluconeogenesis and mobilization of skeletal muscle are essential for providing substrate for the synthesis of acute-phase proteins that are necessary during the various stages of infection. Many of these processes appear to be under the control of interleukin-1.

Recent studies have also identified cachectin as an important control factor. It has been isolated from endotoxin-activated macrophages and has molecular properties similar to interleukin-1. Among cachectin's effects, depression of lipoprotein lipase is important, leading to an abnormal clearance of triglyceride from the circulation. During infection interleukin stimulates the pancreatic cells to release insulin. This probably explains the development of hyperglycaemia and hyperinsulinaemia during systemic infection. It is claimed that interleukin and cachectin are responsible for weight loss during chronic infection, but the evidence supporting this is not conclusive.

It has been demonstrated that fasting *per se* can be responsible for the malabsorption of sugars, amino acids, salt and water (23) in as few as 3–5 days, and even before histological changes are observed in the intestinal mucosa. The effects of fasting and the diarrhoea associated with it can be cumulative and may lead to severe malnutrition. A direct loss of nutrients into the intestinal lumen may also contribute to a negative nutrient balance during illness; this has been documented particularly with respect to proteins during measles (24) (see below), and most probably also occurs in the case of dysentery accompanied by ulceration.

The intestinal mucosa is made up of cells that are produced and, usually within a few days, shed into the lumen where they are broken down and nutrients are released. There is thus a continual enteral-systemic circulation of endogenous nutrients, which are lost as a result of accelerated gastrointestinal transit that is characteristic of diarrhoeal diseases. In health, these nutrients are well absorbed and faecal losses are minimal. During infection, however, there may be increased losses and/or poor absorption. Any cause of intestinal damage is likely to lead to increased rates of shedding.

Furthermore, there may be increased permeability of the intestinal mucosa allowing leakage of endogenous nutrients between the intestinal cells (25). In addition, certain parasites may cause microscopic blood losses. Changes in intestinal permeability have been clearly demonstrated in children with diarrhoea in the Gambia. Interestingly, there are also marked changes in intestinal permeability during severe systemic infections such as measles. This may be accompanied by considerable losses of α_1-antitrypsin in the stool suggesting major losses of endogenous nutrients (25). If the absorptive mechanisms are intact and the damage is in the upper intestine, much of this nutrient leakage will be re-absorbed. If the damage is below the maximally absorptive area of the intestine, however, there will be considerable nutrient losses via the faeces.

The pathophysiological mechanisms by which infectious processes may have a harmful effect on nutritional status may be compounded by the intentional reduction of a child's food intake decided by the mother or other person in charge. This practice is associated with a common belief in most cultures— unfortunately supported by many physicians—that dietary restrictions are beneficial during periods of disease.

The presence of undigested foods or an excess of fat in the stool is also frequently interpreted as a valid reason for limiting a child's food intake. This practice persists despite studies (20) demonstrating that the essential point under these circumstances is not stool composition but what is retained by the body. Thus, even in severe cases where up to 30–40% of ingested nutrients are lost through the faeces, it is important to recall that 60–70% are still absorbed and utilized.

Increased metabolic demands

In addition to reduced food intake and nutrient absorption, nutritional demands are higher during periods of infectious diseases. These demands are linked in varying degrees, as a function of the nature and stage of development of the infective process, to the following factors:

— increased energy needs in the presence of fever;
— increased anabolism for the synthesis of defensive tissues and substances, for example lymphocytes and immunoglobulins;
— increased catabolism resulting from tissue destruction during the acute stage of infection;
— higher nutrient needs for use in tissue reconstruction during recovery. The net result may be a negative nutrient balance during the acute stage, which may be prolonged during convalescence if not corrected by adequate nutrient intake.

General infections

Prospective studies of growth and morbidity in children have identified certain infections as particularly important where poor growth is concerned, e.g., diarrhoeal and respiratory infections and malaria, which are the most prevalent. The impact of infection on growth varies according to a child's nutritional status; food availability (its texture, bulkiness and the time to prepare and feed); cultural beliefs; and access to health care facilities (26).

Diarrhoeal diseases

For children with mild forms of diarrhoea without dehydration, the usual diet may be maintained or should be corrected if it is insufficient; no dietary restrictions are indicated, even for short periods. For severe cases, the child's usual diet and age will determine the appropriate dietary management during periods of infection. The following examples are considered below: infants who are exclusively breast-fed; infants who are fed on breast-milk substitutes, with or without breast milk; and infants and young children who are fed on a mixed diet. Finally, brief consideration is given to nutritional requirements during convalescence.

Infants who are exclusively breast-fed. As noted in chapter 2, infants who are exclusively breast-fed are at much lower risk from diarrhoeal diseases (27) owing to the combined effect of reduced exposure to infective agents and the protective properties of human milk. However, these infants can develop diarrhoeal infections, particularly those of viral origin (see chapter 3). In such cases, as with patients of any age and habitual diet, the prevention of dehydration and electrolyte imbalance, or their correction if already present, is the first priority. These infants should be managed by increasing the frequency of breast-feeding (28).

A recent study (29) compared the effect of interrupting or maintaining breast-feeding during the initial 24 hours of oral rehydration therapy. Infants who were breast-fed during the early phase of acute diarrhoea had fewer, and a smaller volume of, diarrhoeal stools; they required less oral rehydration fluid; and they recovered from diarrhoea sooner than those infants for whom breast-feeding was interrupted. The benefits of breast-feeding appear to be related to the presence in the intestinal lumen of the products of breast-milk digestion (amino acids, dipeptides and hexoses), which may enhance the absorption of sodium and water, thereby reducing the frequency and volume of stools. Breast-feeding thus appears to be beneficial both nutritionally and in terms of the clinical outcome of the diarrhoeal episode.

There is some risk of hypernatraemia when oral rehydration salts are given to small infants (30), particularly those fed with breast-milk substitutes having a high sodium content, but recent studies suggest that it is minimal (31). The risk is reduced when breast-feeding is continued during the diarrhoea, thanks to breast milk's low sodium content and the small amount of oral rehydration solution that is required in these circumstances.

Infants who are fed on breast-milk substitutes. In contrast, bottle-fed infants and children receiving foods other than milk, particularly in an unsanitary environment, are at much greater risk of infection from contaminated foods and utensils. In the past a common practice for infants who developed diarrhoea while being fed on breast-milk substitutes, whether exclusively or as part of mixed feeding, was to subject them to fasting for 24–48 hours while correcting any dehydration or electrolyte imbalances. Infant formula was subsequently reintroduced, beginning with a half-strength dilution fed in small quantities and progressively increasing the concentration and amount until the feeding schedule prior to the episode was reached within 3–5 days. At the same time, breast-feeding was frequently discontinued.

The rationale for this approach was to give the gastrointestinal tract time to "rest" while rehydration was being carried out intravenously. This period was thought to be beneficial for recovering from the anatomical and functional alterations of the intestinal mucosa. It was also assumed that withholding milk was necessary because of the intolerance to lactose and milk proteins that is common during diarrhoea. Moreover, fasting was not difficult to maintain in an anorexic child, who may also have been vomiting. This practice was developed on clinical grounds in the absence of objective experimental demonstrations of its advantages over other feeding schedules. The demonstrated effectiveness of oral rehydration therapy has led in recent years to a reconsideration of the whole issue of dietary management of children during diarrhoea.

Fasting has a negative impact on children's nutritional status, particularly if they are already malnourished. If recommended by a health worker, this practice may also reinforce a mother's belief about the danger of feeding a child who has diarrhoea. The fasting period could well be prolonged beyond the recommended time, with further harmful consequences for the child's nutritional status. Not only has it been demonstrated that fasting is not beneficial, but also that it may well have a highly negative effect on the concentration of intestinal enzymes. This is significant since the presence of substrates in the intestinal lumen stimulates recovery from temporary enzyme deficiencies (*32*).

Intolerance to lactose and milk proteins during diarrhoea has been known for many years to be a physiopathological manifestation of diarrhoea that has to be overcome (*33*). Feeding children under these circumstances does not necessarily cause fur-

ther damage, however. Recent controlled studies (*34–37*) suggest that the feeding of full-strength milk can be resumed after a period of no more than 6–8 hours, during which time the children are being rehydrated, or should not be interrupted at all if they are not dehydrated and maintain a good appetite. Vomiting was frequently observed, but was not severe enough to justify a change in diet. Correction of dehydration and electrolyte imbalance, which is usually accompanied by appetite recovery, seems to be essential for the rapid reintroduction of full-strength milk. If children are not fully rehydrated and remain anorexic, the forcing of full-strength milk may result in acidosis, which only aggravates vomiting.

It is important to note that the studies in question were carried out among essentially well-nourished infants who were suffering from mild forms of diarrhoea lasting only a few days. Caution is still required during the first stages of diarrhoea, particularly in very severe cases and when infants are undernourished. Further studies are required, especially with regard to the influence of different etiologies. However, available evidence indicates that, with appropriate initial correction of dehydration, infants fed with breast-milk substitutes can rapidly be put back onto their pre-diarrhoea diet, and that there is no need for long and dangerous fasting periods. Some dilution of initial feeds would probably be convenient, and rice water has been found to be particularly well-suited for this purpose. The use of cereal products mixed with infant formula may also be beneficial, particularly if children are at an age when complementary feeding is nutritionally required.

In any case, there is no justification at all for interrupting breast-feeding, even for a few hours, when children are receiving breast-milk substitutes. On the contrary, the best course of action for a sick child would be to increase breast-milk intake in order to replace entirely any substitute that is being given.

Children fed on a mixed diet. Infants and young children who are already receiving a mixed and varied diet, including solid foods, are also frequently subjected to severe dietary restrictions when suffering from diarrhoea. Milk and solid foods – typically those with the highest nutritional value – are often withheld entirely, and dietary intake is limited to tea, rice water or thin starchy gruels. Even though such dietary restrictions may be recommended for only a few days, it is not unusual for a mother to prolong them with potentially serious consequences, both for the evolution of the diarrhoea and her child's nutritional status.

It has been demonstrated in controlled studies

(34, 35), however, that rapid re-feeding of the child, using the habitual diet after only a few hours of oral rehydration therapy, does not worsen the child's condition or increase the risk of complications. On the contrary, this approach shortens the duration of diarrhoea and the length of hospital stay, and results in less weight loss and a quicker improvement in the child's general well-being. It appears that good initial rehydration and correction of electrolyte imbalances, which usually result in appetite recovery, are essential for successful and rapid reintroduction of the child's habitual diet.

These observations were made in industrialized countries in cases of acute diarrhoea, most of which could be classified as mild and of less than seven days' duration. The infants in question had most probably gone through a period of dietary restrictions before coming to hospital, and their intakes were the established low-residue and high nutritional value diets of the majority of young children in industrialized countries.

In a similar study conducted in Indonesia (38), children suffering from diarrhoea, some of them malnourished, were put back onto their full previous diet in a progressive but rapid manner within 2–4 days. This contrasted with the 9–11 days for the controls, which was the conventional approach in the environment in question. There was no difference between the two groups in duration of diarrhoea, and those children who underwent rapid re-feeding performed better in terms of weight gain, suggesting that the observations made above in regard to industrialized countries are valid everywhere.

This conclusion is of considerable importance given the high incidence of diarrhoeal and other infectious diseases in developing countries and the degree to which related prolonged dietary restrictions aggravate the already poor nutritional status of so many young children, who in turn may fail to recuperate their losses during convalescence due to an absence of nutritious high-energy foods. It is therefore essential that these observations be repeated under the conditions, including the diets, prevailing in these countries. The foods that are frequently available to young children in this environment, for example starchy roots and tubers, non-refined cereals, leguminous seeds and leafy vegetables, are characterized by their low energy concentration, high fibre content and poor digestibility. Finding out how children with diarrhoea react to rapid re-feeding with these types of foods, or to an appropriate selection from among them, or to their modification to make them more easily digestible and increase their energy density, is of potentially immense value for the health of this group.

Other diseases

There are fewer controlled studies on the dietary management of other infectious diseases than on the management of diarrhoeal diseases. However, there is no reason to suspect that the principles discussed above with respect to diarrhoeal diseases would not apply to other acute infections. Where diet is concerned, the child's appetite is the best guide. Small amounts of favourite nutritious foods should be offered frequently.

Children with high fevers are usually anorexic and will vomit easily; it is not recommended, therefore, that they be forced to eat. Reduction of fever by tepid sponging and relief of pain by appropriate nursing care, topical treatment (such as gentian violet to *Monilia* buccal lesions) and analgesics are all important in the nutritional management of infection. Adequate treatment of the disease itself and prevention of dehydration have first priority; the result should be a prompt return of appetite, thereby permitting normal feeding and improvement in overall health status. As in the case of diarrhoeal diseases, the period of convalescence provides an important opportunity to compensate for nutritional losses incurred and to correct possible deficiencies in the habitual diet.

Measles. Weight loss during measles has been frequently described. Early studies of measles in West Africa showed considerable weight loss (39) and measles was often reported as the precipitating infection among children with marasmus or kwashiorkor in Nigeria (40). Growth faltering was frequently protracted in Bangladeshi children (41), especially those who developed post-measles dysentery. Indeed, measles appears to be a major crisis in the life of a growing child for several reasons. Not only can it be a severe illness in its own right, but the immune suppression that may persist for three or four months after infection also provides an opportunity for a range of other infections to become established and create their own nutritional problems.

Poor food intake resulting from anorexia, dehydration, fever and buccal lesions, though well recognized by experienced health workers, is poorly documented. There are certain cultural practices whereby food is withdrawn from children as a treatment for measles. The measles virus may damage the intestinal mucosa enough to cause malabsorption and protein loss (42). Severe metabolic disturbances have been documented among Nigerian children during acute measles (43). The rates of whole-body protein synthesis and breakdown are increased, and the latter usually exceeds the former with a net loss of body protein stores. These abnormalities may persist during convalescence.

Studies of energy expenditure among Kenyan children with acute measles show rates during infection that are similar to rates during recovery (44). These results appear to be in conflict with other work which shows that energy expenditure is increased during severe infection. However, the children in the Kenya study were ill for several days and their dietary intake was very low. Consequently, it would be predicted that their energy expenditure would be lower than normal owing to an adaptive response. There is thus a considerable energy gap between intake and expenditure during severe measles.

Malaria. The impact of malaria on nutritional status varies according to age, immunological status and intensity of infection. There are important effects on birth weight and the neonate's iron and folate status (45), while impaired growth and anaemia may occur among older children and adolescents. Equally important, however, is immune suppression permitting the development of other infections, which themselves may lead to malnutrition.

Respiratory infections. Although studies in the Gambia (46) and Guatemala (47) show an association between various respiratory infections and faltering growth, there is little information on the relevant cause and effect mechanisms. Nevertheless anorexia, fever, pain, vomiting (especially in whooping cough) and associated diarrhoea may all be important contributory factors, particularly in children under one year of age (48).

Intestinal parasites. There are close associations between intestinal parasites and malnutrition. The most prevalent are *Schistosoma*, *Giardia lamblia*, *Ascaris lumbricoides*, hookworm, *Trichuris trichiura* and *Strongyloides stercoralis*, and several recent reviews have concentrated on intestinal abnormalities (49, 50) and systemic effects (51). There are several problems in assessing the impact of intestinal parasites. For example, there is increasing evidence that, for some parasites at least, there are individuals who have particularly high worm loads. Unless this fact is taken into account during intervention studies, it may be difficult to assess the impact of a community de-worming programme.

Ascaris. Successful de-worming in ascariasis has produced different nutritional effects in different studies. For example, the de-worming of Indian children resulted in a small but significant improvement in weight for age (52). The situation was similar among Kenyan children (53), while Tanzanian chil-

dren (54), who received levamisole every three months, demonstrated quite striking rates of weight gain. In contrast, a study among Ethiopian children failed to show weight gain or enlargement of the mid-upper arm circumference following treatment with piperazine (55).

Studies in Guatemala (56) and Bangladesh (57) have sometimes been quoted as showing no impact of de-worming on growth, although worms were not in fact successfully eliminated in either case. Studies in Papua New Guinea (58) and Brazil (59) showed no significant impact of de-worming on nutritional status, but then the children in question were relatively well nourished to begin with.

Schistosoma. Different nutritional problems are linked to different species. For example, *Schistosoma haematobium* is associated with thinness, as in the case of a low body-mass index noted in Nigerian boys who were thus infected (60). Similarly, there was improvement in a range of anthropometric indices among a group of Kenyan children with *S. haematobium* following metrifonate therapy (61). The mechanisms for growth impairment have not been studied, but it is interesting that animals having schistosomiasis experience anorexia (62). *S. mansoni* is associated with anaemia and poor growth, sometimes with a decrease in plasma proteins and low ferritin levels (63). However, there appears to be no study in which the impact of de-worming on nutritional status has been assessed. The association between *S. japonicum* and malnutrition (both stunting and anaemia) are well described (64), but there are no data on how these features change after de-worming.

Hookworm. The iron and protein deficiency resulting from hookworm infection is well known (65). Weight loss is also experienced but unexplained. It has been suggested that anorexia associated with the itching and respiratory symptoms of the infection is important (66).

Trichuris trichiura is rather underestimated as a cause of malnutrition (67), but several studies indicate that it may cause anaemia, weight loss (68) and stunting (67).

Strongyloides stercoralis is associated with anorexia, malabsorption and loss of endogenous nutrients (69). In severe cases there may be subtotal villus atrophy (70), but the nutritional consequences of milder infection are unknown.

Giardia lamblia appears to cause diarrhoea and malabsorption in some subjects more than in others (71). This may be due to differences in immune response to the parasite; the intestinal response to the first exposure appears to be more severe than to subsequent exposure. Studies in Guatemala (72) show that *Giardia* is associated with faltering growth among young, but not among older, children. Longitudinal studies suggest that only some subjects with *Giardia* have any symptoms at all, which has given rise to the suggestion that there may be differences in strain pathogenicity. There is an especially high prevalence of large numbers of *Giardia lamblia* in the upper intestine of children with marasmus or kwashiorkor. Indeed, the presence of *Enterobacteriaceae* in the upper intestine of subjects with *Giardia lamblia* infection may be responsible for the severe degree of malabsorption experienced by some individuals (*73*).

Human immunodeficiency virus (HIV). HIV infection manifests itself in a variety of ways ranging from asymptomatic infection to acquired immunodeficiency syndrome (AIDS) accompanied by life-threatening infections and malignancy (*74–76*). The virus affects the immune system by attacking the lymphocytes and destroying the body's ability to defend itself.

Weight loss or abnormally slow growth, and chronic diarrhoea and prolonged fever (longer than a month) are major signs in infants and children suffering from AIDS (*77*). Of the many consequences of malnutrition, one of the most detrimental is muscle wasting. Heart muscle atrophies and cardiac function is decreased. Starvation may also impair digestion as an indirect result of inadequate pancreatic enzyme production. Deficits of iron, zinc, magnesium, pyridoxine, folate, and vitamins A, C, D and E are known to impair immunity (*78*). (See also the discussion in chapter 3 on HIV infection and breast-feeding.)

Convalescence

The period of convalescence from diarrhoeal and other diseases is characterized by the return of a normal appetite and increased nutritional requirements to permit catch-up growth and the replenishment of nutritional reserves. An ample, balanced diet, rich in the most nutritious foods available, is important since even short periods of disease can seriously affect growth in very young children, and may result in significant weight loss and a depletion of important nutritional reserves of, for example, energy, iron and vitamin A.

Convalescence will thus provide a good opportunity to correct any deficiencies in the habitual diet. It will also be an appropriate time to introduce solid or semi-solid complementary foods to infants who are 4–6 months of age, particularly those who are fed on breast-milk substitutes (see chapter 4). There may well be an important need for micronutrients in pharmacological quantities. For example, there is some suggestion that mortality from measles in children living in a vitamin A-deficient area of the United Republic of Tanzania can be reduced by supplementation with vitamin A (*79*). However, it is not clear as to how much this can be extrapolated to other environments. The fact that mothers may be more receptive to counsel at this juncture, and that their children in turn have good appetites, will help to satisfy increased nutritional requirements and ensure that appropriate feeding practices continue.

A primary requirement is that children receive sufficient dietary energy and nutrients to enable them to achieve their growth potential. In circumstances where there is a considerable weight deficit, requirements will normally be high in order to reduce or abolish it. In an ideal environment there is generally little need to be concerned about catch-up growth. However, in situations where children are subjected to repeated episodes of acute infection, if the catch-up growth between infections is slow, a cumulative deficit builds up (*80*), resulting in increased stunting associated with higher morbidity and mortality.

A satisfactory intake of nutrients may depend on the type of food presented to the child. Such household food technologies as fermentation and germination (*81*) appear to have an important role to play in this regard. Germination decreases the viscosity of food by producing alpha amylases, which hydrolyse starch. In particular, the use of fermented food, a traditional weaning preparation in many societies, may have considerable advantages both in terms of inhibiting the growth of pathogens and because of its taste, increased energy density and digestibility (*81*).

Résumé

Le nourrisson et le jeune enfant au cours des infections aiguës

L'immunité passive conférée par les anticorps et le lait maternel protège l'enfant contre l'infection durant les premiers mois de la vie. C'est durant le deuxième semestre que les risques infectieux et notamment de survenue de maladies diarrhéiques augmentent le plus rapidement. Après 3 ans en général l'incidence des infections décroît. Pour les enfants qui n'ont pas reçu le sein les risques sont plus grands et aussi plus précoces. Dans l'ensemble, il est difficile de faire la part de ce qui revient à l'infection et à la malnutrition dans les retards de croissance que l'on peut observer à la longue, car il existe une synergie entre les deux.

Les effets de l'infection sur l'état nutritionnel et les mécanismes qui aboutissent à la malnutrition sont présentés. L'anorexie en premier, qui accompagne les maladies infectieuses est l'un de ces mécanismes et ne semble pas causée directement par la fièvre. C'est l'interleukine 1 libérée par les macrophages qui semble être le médiateur. De même la carence en fer a été associée à une diminution de l'immunité cellulaire et de l'activité bactéricide augmentant la prévalence des infections respiratoires et de la diarrhée. A l'opposé cependant l'injection parentérale de fortes doses de fer augmente les taux d'infections. La diminution de l'apport alimentaire entraînant la diminution d'apport en fer et probablement en autres ions pourrait alors être considérée comme un moyen de défense. Les vomissements ainsi que les moniliases buccales peuvent aussi limiter les apports.

En second lieu interviennent les perturbations de l'absorption intestinale et les pertes en nutriments par voie digestive. La malabsorption n'est pas préoccupante au cours d'un épisode infectieux unique mais elle a un retentissement significatif sur le statut nutritionnel quand les épisodes se prolongent et surtout quand ils se répètent. L'infection entraîne des réponses métaboliques variées qui retentissent sur l'utilisation des aliments et la mobilisation des réserves corporelles. L'interleukine 1 semble contrôler certains des processus qui conduisent à la néoglucogenèse et à la mobilisation des protéines musculaires. La cachexine apparaît être aussi un élément de contrôle important. Des besoins nutritionnels accrus viennent s'ajouter à la réduction des apports et aux troubles de l'absorption à cause d'une demande énergétique plus grande liée à la fièvre, d'une augmentation des synthèses au niveau des systèmes de défense, d'un catabolisme accéléré de tous les tissus et d'un besoin plus grand en nutriments pour compenser ce catabolisme.

Des enquêtes prospectives ont montré que certaines infections ont un impact important sur la croissance et la morbidité des enfants notamment la diarrhée, les infections respiratoires et le paludisme. Il faut insister sur le fait que le régime alimentaire habituel doit être maintenu sans aucune interruption dans le cas de diarrhées modérées sans déshydratation. Les enfants nourris au sein peuvent développer des diarrhées sévères d'origine virale particulièrement et les sels de réhydratation doivent être administrés sans interrompre l'allaitement maternel, le risque d'hypernatrémie étant minime; chez les enfants nourris artificiellement, pour lesquels les risques sont plus importants, les mises à la diète pendant 24 ou 48 heures, prescrites traditionnellement, sont inutiles et leurs effets négatifs sont parfaitement documentés; enfin les enfants dont l'alimentation est diversifiée bénéficient eux aussi de la réinstallation rapide d'un régime normal après quelques heures de réhydratation.

Il existe moins d'enquêtes contrôlées sur les conduites diététiques à observer dans d'autres maladies infectieuses que pour les maladies diarrhéiques. Il n'y a cependant pas de raison pour que les principes décrits ne s'appliquent pas aux infections comme la rougeole, le paludisme, les infections respiratoires, les parasitoses intestinales; il faut signaler le syndrome d'immunodéficience acquise (SIDA) qui s'accompagne d'une maigreur importante entraînée par la malabsorption et la malnutrition.

La convalescence d'une diarrhée ou d'une autre maladie infectieuse est caractérisée par le retour à un appétit normal et à des besoins nutritionnels accrus pour la reprise de la croissance et la reconstitution des réserves.

References

1. **Hanson, L.A. et al.** Immune response in the mammary gland. In: Ogra, P.L. & Dayton, D.H., ed. *Immunology of breast milk.* New York, Raven Press, 1979, p. 145.

2. **Sahni, S. & Chandra, R.K.** Malnutrition and susceptibility to diarrhoea, with special reference to the anti-infective properties of breast milk. In: Chen, L.C. & Scrimshaw, N.S., ed. *Diarrhoea and malnutrition.* New York, Plenum Press, 1983, p. 99.

3. **Gordon, J.E. et al.** Weanling diarrhea. *Am. j. med. sci.*, **245**: 345–377 (1963).

4. **Mata, L.J. & Urrutia, J.J.** Intestinal colonization of breast-fed children in a rural area of low socioeconomic level. *Ann. N.Y. Acad. Sci.*, **176**: 93–109 (1971).

5. **Dyson, T.** Levels, trends, differentials and causes of child mortality. A survey. *Wld hlth stat. rep.*, **30**: 282–311 (1977).

6. **Feachem, R.G. & Koblinsky, M.A.** Interventions for the control of diarrhoeal diseases among young children: promotion of breast-feeding. *Bull. Wld Hlth Org.*, **62**: 271–291 (1984).

7. **Scrimshaw, N.S. et al.** *Interaction of nutrition and infection.* Geneva, World Health Organization, 1968. (WHO Monograph Series No. 57).

8. **Rowland, M.G.M. et al.** Impact of infection on the growth of children from 0 to 2 years in an urban West African community. *Am. j. clin. nutr.*, **47**: 134–138 (1988).

9. **Zumrawi, F.Y. et al.** Effects of infection on growth in Sudanese children. *Human nutrition*, **41C**: 453–461 (1987).

10. The nutritional consequences of acute and chronic infections. In: Protein-energy requirements under conditions prevailing in developing countries: current knowledge and research needs. The United Nations University World Hunger Programme, *Food and nutrition bulletin* (*supplement 1*): 24–33 (1979).

11. **McCarthy, I.O. et al.** The role of fever in appetite suppression after endotoxin administration. *Am. j. clin. nutr.*, **40**: 310–316 (1984).

12. **Baile, C.A. et al.** Endotoxin-elicited fever and anorexia and elfazepam-stimulated feeding in sheep. *Physio. behav.*, **27**: 271–277 (1981).

13. **Keusch, G.T. & Farthing, M.J.G.** Nutrition and infection. *Ann. rev. nutr.*, **6**: 131–154 (1986).

14. **Golden, M.H.N. & Ramdath, D.** Free radicals in the pathogenesis of kwashiorkor. *Proc. Nutr. Soc.*, **46**: 53–68 (1987).

15. **Basta, S.S. et al.** Iron deficiency anaemia and the productivity of adult males in Indonesia. *Am. j. clin. nutr.*, **32**: 916–925 (1979).

16. **Oppenheimer, S.J. et al.** Effect of iron prophylaxis on morbidity due to infectious disease: report on clinical studies in Papua New Guinea. *Transact. Roy. Soc. Trop. Med.* **80**: 596–602 (1986).

17. **Martorell, R. et al.** The impact of ordinary illnesses on the dietary intakes of malnourished children. *Am. j. clin. nutr.*, **33**: 345–350 (1980).

18. **Hoyle, B. et al.** Breast-feeding and food intake among children with acute diarrheal disease. *Am. j. clin. nutr.*, **33**: 2365–2371 (1980).

19. **Molla, A.M. et al.** Food intake during and after recovery from diarrhoea in children. In: Chen, L.C. & Scrimshaw, N.S., ed. *Diarrhoea and malnutrition.* New York, Plenum Press, 1983, pp. 113–123.

20. **Chung, A.W.** The effect of oral feeding at different levels on the absorption of foodstuffs in infantile diarrhoea. *J. pediatr.*, **33**: 1–13 (1948).

21. **Molla, A.M. et al.** Effects of acute diarrhoea on absorption of macronutrients during disease and after recovery. In: Chen, L.C. & Scrimshaw, N.S., ed. *Diarrhoea and malnutrition.* New York, Plenum Press, 1983, p. 143.

22. **Tomkins, A.M.** Tropical malabsorption: recent concepts in pathogenesis and nutritional significance. *Clinical science*, **60**: 131–137 (1981).

23. **Billich, C. et al.** Absorptive capacity of the jejunum of obese and lean subjects. Effects of fasting. *Arch. internat. med.*, **130**: 377–380 (1972).

24. **Axton, J.H.M.** Measles: a protein-losing enteropathy. *Br. med. j.*, **3**: 79–80 (1974).

25. **Behrens, R.H. et al.** Factors affecting the integrity of the intestinal mucosa of Gambian infants. *Am. j. clin. nutr.*, **45**: 1433–1441 (1987).

26. **Tomkins, A.M.** Improving nutrition in developing countries. Can primary health care help? *Trop. med. parasitol.*, **38**: 226–232 (1987).

27. **Victora, C.G. et al.** Evidence for protection by breast-feeding against infant deaths from infectious diseases in Brazil. *Lancet*, **2**: 319–321 (1987).

28. *The treatment and prevention of acute diarrhoea: practical guidelines.* 2nd ed. Geneva, World Health Organization, 1989.

29. **Khing-Maung, U. et al.** Effect on clinical outcome of breast-feeding during acute diarrhoea. *Br. med. j.*, **290**: 587–589 (1985).

30. **Clary, T.G. et al.** The relationship of oral rehydration solution to hypernatremia in infantile diarrhoea. *J. pediatr.*, **99**: 739–741 (1981).

31. **Helmy, N. et al.** Oral rehydration therapy for low-birth-weight neonates suffering from diarrhoea in the intensive-care unit. *J. paed. gastroenterol. nutr.*, **7**: 417–423 (1988).

32. **Pergolizzi, R.F. et al.** Interaction between dietary carbohydrates and intestinal disaccharidases in experimental diarrhoea. *Am. j. clin. nutr.*, **30**: 482–489 (1977).

33. **Ianow, D.C.** Nutritional disturbances. In: Holt, L.E. et al., ed. *Pediatrics.* 13th ed. New York, Century-Crofts, 1962, p. 229.

34. **Isolauri, E. et al.** Milk versus no milk in rapid re-feeding after acute gastroenteritis. *J. ped. gastroenterol. nutr.*, **5**: 254–261 (1986).

35. **Dugdale, A. et al.** Re-feeding after acute gastroenteritis: a controlled study. *Arch. dis. child.*, **57**: 76–78 (1982).

36. **Rees, L. & Brook, C.G.D.** Gradual reintroduction of full-strength milk after acute gastroenteritis in children. *Lancet*, **1**: 770–771 (1979).

37. **Placzek, M. & Walter-Smith, J.A.** Comparison of two feeding regimens following acute gastroenteritis in infancy. *J. ped. gastroenterol. nutr.*, **3**: 245–248 (1984).

38. **Soeprapto et al.** Feeding children with diarrhoea. *J. trop. ped. and environm. child hlth*, **25**: 97–100 (1979).

39. **Morley, D.** Severe measles in the tropics. *Br. med. j.*, **1**: 297–300 (1969).

40. **Laditan, A.A.O. & Reeds, P.J.** A study of the age of onset, diet and the importance of infection in the pattern of severe protein-energy malnutrition in Ibadan, Nigeria. *Br. j. nutr.*, **36**: 411–419 (1976).

41. **Koster, F.T. et al.** Synergistic impact of measles and diarrhoea on nutrition and mortality in Bangladesh. *Bull. Wld Hlth Org.*, **59**: 901–908 (1981).

42. **Dosseter, J.F.B. & Whittle, H.C.** Protein-losing enteropathy and malabsorption in acute measles enteritis. *Br. med. j.*, **2**: 592–593 (1975).

43. **Tomkins, A.M. et al.** The combined effects of infection and malnutrition on protein metabolism in children. *Clin. sci.*, **65**: 313–324 (1983).

44. **Duggan, M.B. & Milner, R.D.G.** Composition of weight gain by Kenyan children during recovery from measles. *Hum. nutr. clin. nutr.*, **40C**: 173–183 (1986).

45. **Fleming, A.F. et al.** The prevention of anaemia in pregnancy in primigravidae in the guinea savanna of Nigeria. *Ann. trop. med. parasitol.*, **80**: 211–233 (1987).

46. **Rowland, M.G.M. et al.** A quantitative study into the role of infection in determining nutritional status in Gambian village children. *Br. j. nutr.*, **37**: 441–450 (1977).

47. **Mata, L.J. et al.** Effect of infection on food intake and the nutritional state: perspectives as viewed from the village. *Am. j. clin. nutr.*, **30**: 1215–1227 (1977).

48. **Eylenbosch, W. & Tanner, J.** *Child mortality and growth in a small African town: a longitudinal study of 6228 children from Kasongo (Zaire).* Antwerp, Institute of Tropical Medicine, 1987, pp. 171–191.

49. **Stephenson, L.S.** *Impact of helminth infections on human nutrition.* London, Taylor & Francis, 1987.

50. **Hall, A.** Nutritional aspects of parasitic infection. *Prog. food. nutr. sci.*, **9**: 227–256 (1985).

51. **Tomkins, A.M.** The interaction of parasitic diseases and nutrition. *Pontificiae Academiae Scientiarum Scripta Varia*, **61**: 23–43 (1985).

52. **Gupta, M.C. et al.** Effect of periodic de-worming on nutritional status of *Ascaris*-infected preschool children receiving supplementary food. *Lancet*, **2**: 108–110 (1977).

53. **Stephenson, L.S. et al.** Relationships between *Ascaris* infection and growth of malnourished preschool children in Kenya. *Am. j. clin. nutr.*, **33**: 1165–1172 (1980).

54. **Willett, W.C. et al.** *Ascaris* and growth rates: a randomized trial of treatment. *Am. J. pub. hlth*, **69**: 987–991 (1979).

55. **Freij, L. et al.** Ascariasis and malnutrition. A study in urban Ethiopian children. *Am. j. clin. nutr.*, **32**: 1545–1553 (1979).

56. **Gupta, M.C. & Urrutia, J.J.** Effect of periodic antiascaris and antigiardia treatment on nutritional status of preschool children. *Am. j. clin. nutr.*, **36**: 79–86 (1982).

57. **Greenberg, B.L. et al.** Single dose piperazine therapy for *Ascaris lumbricoides*: an unsuccessful method of promoting growth. *Am. j. clin. nutr.*, **34**: 2508–2516 (1981).

58. **Pust, R.E. et al.** Palm oil and pyrantel as child nutrition mass interventions in Papua New Guinea. *Trop. geog. med.*, **37**: 1–10 (1985).

59. **Kloetzel, K. et al.** Ascariasis and malnutrition in a group of Brazilian children—a follow-up study. *J. trop. paedatr.*, **28**: 41–43 (1982).

60. **Oomen, J.M.V. et al.** Difference in blood status of three ethnic groups inhabiting the same locality in northern Nigeria: anaemia, splenomegaly and associated causes. *Trop. geog. med.*, **31**: 587–606 (1979).

61. **Stephenson, L.S. et al.** Relationships of *Schistosoma haematobium*, hookworm and malarial infections and metrifonate treatment to growth of Kenyan schoolchildren. *Am. j. trop. med. hyg.*, **34**: 1109–1118 (1985).

62. **Cheever, A.W.** *Schistosoma haematobium*: the pathology of experimental infection. *Exp. parasitol.*, **59**: 131–138 (1985).

63. **Mansour, M.M. et al.** Prevalence of latent iron deficiency in patients with chronic *S. mansoni* infection. *Trop. geog. med.*, **37**: 124–128 (1985)

64. **Horn, J.S.** Death to the snails! The fight against schistosomiasis. In: *Away with all pests: an English surgeon in People's China 1954–1969*. New York, Monthly Review Press, 1969.

65. **Gilles, H.M. et al.** Hookworm infection and anaemia. *Q. j. med.*, **33**: 1–24 (1964).

66. **Latham, M.C.** Needed research on the interactions of certain parasitic diseases and nutrition in humans. *Rev. infect. dis.*, **4**: 896–900 (1982).

67. **Cooper, E.S. & Bundy, D.A.P.** Trichuris is not trivial. *Parasitol. today*, **4**: 301–306 (1988).

68. **Cooper, E.S. & Bundy, D.A.P.** Trichuriasis in Saint Lucia. In: McNeish, A.S. & Walker-Smith, J.A., ed. *Diarrhoea and malnutrition in children*. London, Butterworths, 1986.

69. **O'Brien, W.** Intestinal malabsorption in acute infection with *Strongyloides stercoralis*. *Trans. Roy. Soc. Trop. Med. Hyg.*, **69**: 69–77 (1975).

70. **Tomkins, A.M.** The role of intestinal parasites in diarrhoea and malnutrition. *Trop. doctor*, **9**: 21–24 (1979).

71. **Wright, S.G. et al.** Giardiasis: clinical and therapeutic aspects. *Gut*, **18**: 343–350 (1977).

72. **Farthing, M.J.G. et al.** Natural history of *Giardia* infection of infants and children in rural Guatemala and its impact on physical growth. *Am. j. clin. nutr.*, **43**: 395–405 (1986).

73. **Tomkins, A.M. et al.** Bacterial colonization of jejunal mucosa in giardiasis. *Trans. Roy. Soc. Trop. Med. Hyg.*, **72**: 33–36 (1978).

74. **Center for Diseases Control.** Revision of the CDC surveillance case definition for acquired immunodeficiency syndrome. *J. Am. Med. Assoc.*, **258**: 1143–1154 (1987).

75. **Gottlieb, M.S. et al.** The acquired immunodeficiency syndrome. *Ann. intern. med.*, **99**: 208–220 (1983).

76. **Fauci, A.S. et al.** Acquired immunodeficiency syndrome: epidemiologic, clinical, immunologic, and therapeutic considerations. *Ann. intern. med.*, **100**: 92–108 (1984).

77. **Colebunders, G.A. et al.** Evaluation of a clinical case definition of AIDS in African children. *AIDS*, **1**: 151–156 (1987).

78. **Bentler, M. & Stanish, M.** Nutrition support of the pediatric patient with AIDS. *J. Am. Diet. Assoc.*, **87**: 488–491 (1987).

79. **Barclay, A.J.G. et al.** Vitamin A supplements and mortality related to measles. *Br. med. j.*, **294**: 294–296 (1987).

80. Nutrient requirements for catch-up growth and tissue repletion. In: Protein-energy requirements under conditions prevailing in developing countries: current knowledge and research needs. The United Nations University World Hunger Programme, *Food and nutrition bulletin*, (Supplement 1): 34–48 (1979).

81. *Proceedings of a UNICEF/Swedish International Development Authority Workshop on Household Technologies for Improved Weaning Foods, Nairobi, October 1987*, New York, UNICEF, 1988.

Check-list for evaluating the adequacy of support for breast-feeding in maternity hospitals, wards and clinics

In 1989 the World Health Organization and the United Nations Children's Fund (UNICEF) issued a joint statement[a] on the role of maternity services in protecting, promoting and supporting breast-feeding. Taking into consideration the community attitudes that variously sustain or restrain breast-feeding, the statement translates the most up-to-date scientific knowledge and practical experience about lactation into precise, universally applicable, recommendations on care for mothers before, during and after pregnancy and delivery. Information is addressed to health workers, particularly clinicians, midwives and nursing personnel, but also to policy-makers and managers of maternal and child health and family planning facilities. The statement concludes with a 20-point synthesis in the form of a check-list (see below), which can be used in maternity wards and clinics to gauge how well they are promoting and supporting breast-feeding. The check-list is intended to be a suggestive rather than exhaustive inventory of the kinds of practical steps that can be taken within and through maternity services. Under ideal circumstances, the answers to all the questions will be "yes". A negative reply may indicate an inappropriate practice that should be modified in accordance with the WHO/UNICEF recommendations.

Policy

1. Does the health care facility have an explicit policy for protecting, promoting and supporting breast-feeding?
2. Is this policy communicated to those responsible for managing and providing maternity services (for example in oral briefings when new staff are employed; in manuals, guidelines and other written materials; or by supervisory personnel)?
3. Is there a mechanism for evaluating the effectiveness of the breast-feeding policy? For example:
   - Are data being collected on the prevalence of breast-feeding initiation and breast-feeding at the time of discharge of mothers and their infants from the health care facility?
   - Is there a system for assessing related health

[a] Protecting, promoting and supporting breast-feeding: The special role of maternity services. A Joint WHO/UNICEF Statement. World Health Organization 1989, iv+32 pages. ISBN 92 4 156130 0

Language editions available or in preparation: Arabic, Bengali, Catalan, Chinese, Czech, Danish, Dutch, English, Farsi, French, German, Greek, Hungarian, Bahasa Indonesia, Italian, Kannada, Korean, Malay, Nepali, Oriya, Polish, Portuguese, Russian, Serbo-Croatian, Sindhi, Slovak, Spanish, Swedish, Thai, Turkish, Ukranian, Vietnamese

Liste de contrôle pour déterminer le degré d'adéquation du soutien apporté à l'allaitement maternel dans les hôpitaux, maternités et cliniques

En 1989, l'Organisation mondiale de la Santé et le Fonds des Nations Unies pour l'enfance (UNICEF) ont publié une déclaration conjointe[a] sur le rôle des services liés à la maternité dans la protection, l'encouragement et le soutien de l'allaitement maternel. Tenant compte des attitudes de la communauté en général qui encouragent ou dissuadent l'allaitement maternel, la déclaration traduit les connaissances scientifiques les plus actuelles et l'expérience pratique de la lactation en recommandations précises sur les soins à apporter aux mères avant, pendant et après la grossesse et l'accouchement. Cette information s'adresse aux personnels de santé, particulièrement aux médecins practiciens, aux sages-femmes et au personnel infirmier, mais aussi aux décideurs et aux gestionnaires des services de santé maternelle et infantile et de planning familial. La déclaration s'achève par une synthèse en 20 points (voir ci-dessous) que les services liés à la maternité peuvent utiliser pour évaluer la manière dont ils encouragent et soutiennent l'allaitement maternel. Cette liste est conçue comme un inventaire indicatif plutôt qu'exhaustif des mesures pratiques qui peuvent être prises dans les établissements de soins. Dans les circonstances idéales la réponse à toutes les questions de la liste sera "oui". Une réponse négative peut traduire une démarche qui ne convient pas et qu'il faudrait modifier conformément aux recommandations de l'OMS et de l'UNICEF.

Principes directeurs

1. L'établissement de soins a-t-il une politique explicite de protection, d'encouragement et de soutien de l'allaitement maternel?
2. Cette politique est-elle portée à la connaissance des gestionnaires et des prestateurs de soins (lors de séances d'information orale au moment du recrutement de personnel nouveau, sous la forme de manuels, directives ou autre documentation écrite, ou encore par le personnel d'encadrement)?
3. Existe-t-il un système pour évaluer l'efficacité de la politique en matière d'allaitement maternel?

[a] Protection, encouragement et soutien de l'allaitement maternel. Le rôle spécial des services liés à la maternité Déclaration conjointe de l'OMS et de l'UNICEF. Organisation mondiale de la Santé, 1989, iv+32 pages, ISBN 92 4 256130 4

Versions disponibles ou en préparation: allemand, anglais, arabe, bengali, catalan, chinois, coréen, danois, espagnol, farsi, français, grec, hongrois, italien, kannada, malais, malais (indonésie), néerlandais, népalais, oriya, polonais, portugais, russe, serbo-croate, sindhi, slovaque, suédois, tchèque, thaï, turc, ukrainien, vietnamien.

care practices and training and promotional materials, including those commonly used by antenatal and postnatal services?

4. Are the cooperation and support of all interested parties, particularly health care providers, breast-feeding counsellors and mothers' support groups, but also the general public, sought in developing and implementing the health care facility's breast-feeding policy?

Staff training

5. Are all health care staff well aware of the importance and advantages of breast-feeding and acquainted with the health care facility's policy and services to protect, promote and support breast-feeding?
6. Has the health care facility provided specialized training in lactation management to specific staff members?

Structure and functioning of services

7. Do antenatal records indicate whether breast-feeding has been discussed with a pregnant woman? Is it noted:
   - Whether a woman has indicated her intention to breast-feed?
   - Whether her breasts have been examined?
   - Whether her breast-feeding history has been taken?
   - How long and how often she has already breast-fed?
   - Whether she previously encountered any problems and, if so, what kind?
   - What type of help she received, if any, and from whom?
8. Is a mother's antenatal record available at the time of delivery?
   - If not, is the information in point 7 nevertheless communicated to the staff of the health care facility?
   - Does a woman who has never breast-fed, or who has previously encountered problems with breast-feeding, receive special attention and support from the staff of the health care facility?
9. Does the health care facility take into account a woman's intention to breast-feed when deciding on the use of a sedative, an analgesic or an anaesthetic, if any, during labour and delivery?
   - Are staff familiar with the effects of such medicaments on breast-feeding?
10. In general, are newborn infants:
   - Shown to their mothers within 5 minutes after completion of the second stage of labour?
   - Shown/given to their mothers before silver

Par exemple:
- Cherche-t-on à savoir combien de femmes adoptent l'allaitement au sein et combien le poursuivent à la sortie de l'établissement?
- Existe-t-il un système pour apprécier la pratique des soins et les matériels de formation et de promotion, y compris ceux qui sont couramment utilisés par les services de soins prénatals et postnatals?

4. L'établissement recherche-t-il la coopération et le soutien de toutes les parties intéressées, notamment des prestateurs de soins, des conseillères en allaitement maternel et des associations de soutien aux mères, mais également du public en général, pour l'élaboration et l'application de la politique de l'établissement en matière d'allaitement maternel?

Formation du personnel

5. Tout le personnel soignant est-il au courant de l'importance et des avantages de l'allaitement maternel et informé de la politique et des prestations de l'établissement en vue de protéger, encourager et soutenir la pratique de l'allaitement maternel?
6. L'établissement a-t-il assuré la formation spécialisée de certains membres de son personnel à la "gestion de l'allaitement?"

Structure et fonctionnement des services

7. Les dossiers de soins prénatals indiquent-ils si l'allaitement maternel a fait l'objet d'entretiens avec une femme enceinte?
   Indiquent-ils:
   - Si une femme a fait connaître ou non son intention d'allaiter son enfant au sein?
   - Si elle a fait l'objet d'un examen des seins?
   - Si l'on s'est enquis d'allaitements antérieurs?
   - Si elle a déjà allaité un enfant, combien de fois et pendant combien de temps?
   - Si elle a déjà éprouvé des difficultés, et dans l'affirmative lesquelles?
   - L'aide qu'elle a reçue, le cas échéant, et de qui?
8. L'établissement a-t-il accès, au moment de l'accouchement, au dossier prénatal de la mère?
   - Dans la négative, les indications signalées au point 7 sont-elles quand même communiquées au personnel de l'établissement?
   - Les femmes qui n'ont jamais allaité d'enfant ou qui ont précédemment éprouvé des difficultés d'allaitement bénéficient-elles d'une attention ou d'un soutien spéciaux de la part du personnel de l'établissement?
9. L'établissement tient-il compte de l'intention manifestée par les femmes d'allaiter leur enfant,

nitrate or antibiotic drops are administered prophylactically to the infants' eyes?
- Given to their mothers to hold and put to the breast within a half-hour of completion of the second stage of labour, and allowed to remain with them for at least one hour?

11. Does the health care facility have a rooming-in policy? That is, do infants remain with their mothers throughout their stay?
- Are mothers allowed to have their infants with them in their beds?
- If the infants stay in cots, are these placed close to the mothers' beds?
- If rooming-in applies only during daytime hours, are infants at least brought frequently (every 3–4 hours) to their mothers at night?

12. Is it the health care facility's policy to restrict the giving of prelacteal feeds, that is any food or drink other than breast milk, before breast-feeding has been established?

Health education

13. Are all expectant mothers advised on nutritional requirements during pregnancy and lactation, and on the dangers associated with the use of drugs?

14. Are information and education on breast-feeding routinely provided to pregnant women during antenatal care?

15. Are staff members or counsellors who have specialized training in lactation management available full time to advise breast-feeding mothers during their stay in the health care facility and in preparation for their discharge? Are mothers informed:
- About the physiology of lactation and how to maintain it?
- How to prevent and manage common problems like breast engorgement and sore or cracked nipples?
- Where to turn, for example to breast-feeding support groups, to deal with these or related problems? (Do breast-feeding support groups have access to the health care facility?)

16. Are support and counselling on how to initiate and maintain breast-feeding routinely provided for women who:
- Have undergone Caesarean section?
- Have delivered prematurely?
- Have delivered low-birth-weight infants?
- Have infants who are in special care for any reason?

17. Are breast-feeding mothers provided with printed materials that give relevant guidance and information?

au moment de se prononcer sur l'utilisation d'un sédatif, d'un analgésique ou d'un anesthésique, le cas échéant, durant le travail et l'accouchement?
- Le personnel est-il au courant des effets de ces médicaments sur l'allaitement maternel?

10. En général, les nouveau-nés sont-ils:
- présentés à leur mère dans les cinq minutes suivant la fin de la deuxième phase du travail?
- présentés ou remis à leur mère avant l'administration prophylactique de collyre au nitrate d'argent ou aux antibiotiques?
- remis dans les mains de leur mère et placés au sein dans la demi-heure qui suit l'achèvement de la deuxième phase du travail, et maintenus dans ces conditions pendant au moins une heure?

11. L'établissement a-t-il pour politique d'installer l'enfant dans la chambre de sa mère? C'est-à-dire laisse-t-on les nouveau-nés avec leur mère pendant tout leur séjour?
- Les enfants sont-ils installés dans le lit de leur mère?
- Si les enfants sont placés dans un berceau, le sont-ils à proximité du lit de la mère?
- Si les enfants sont installés dans la chambre de leur mère uniquement durant la journée, sont-ils au moins amenés fréquemment (toutes les trois à quatre heures) à leur mère durant la nuit?

12. L'établissement a-t-il pour politique de limiter au minimum l'administration d'aliments autres que le lait maternel avant le début de l'allaitement au sein?

Education sanitaire

13. Informe-t-on toutes les futures mères des besoins nutritionnels de la grossesse et de la lactation, ainsi que des dangers associés à l'absorption de drogues?

14. Les femmes enceintes reçoivent-elles systématiquement, durant les soins prénatals, des informations et une éducation concernant l'allaitement au sein?

15. Les membres du personnel de l'établissement ou les conseillères qui ont reçu une formation spécialisée à la "gestion de l'allaitement" sont-ils à disposition à plein temps pour conseiller les mères qui allaitent durant leur séjour dans l'établissement et pour les préparer à leur sortie? Les mères sont-elles informées:
- de la physiologie de la lactation et des moyens de l'entretenir?
- de la façon de prévenir ou traiter les problèmes courants tels que l'engorgement des seins ou encore les inflammations ou gerçures des mamelons?

Discharge

18. If "discharge packs" with baby- and personal-care products are provided to mothers when they leave the hospital or clinic, is it the policy of the health care facility to ensure that they contain nothing that might interfere with the successful initiation and establishment of breast-feeding, for example feeding bottles and teats, pacifiers and infant formula?

19. Are mothers or other family members, as appropriate, of infants who are not fed on breast milk given adequate instructions for the correct preparation and feeding of breast-milk substitutes, and a warning against the health hazards of incorrect preparation?
    - Is it the policy of the health care facility not to give such instructions in the presence of breast-feeding mothers?

20. Is every mother given an appointment for her first follow-up visit for postnatal and infant care?
    - Is she informed how to deal with any problems that may arise meanwhile in relation to breast-feeding?

- des associations de soutien à l'allaitement maternel auxquelles s'adresser, par exemple pour traiter ces problèmes ou des problèmes connexes? Ces associations ont-elles leurs entrées dans l'établissement?

16. Offre-t-on systématiquement une aide et des conseils sur la façon d'adopter et de poursuivre l'allaitement au sein aux femmes qui:
    - ont subi une césarienne?
    - ont eu un accouchement prématuré?
    - ont accouché d'un enfant de poids inférieur à la normale?
    - ont eu un enfant qui doit recevoir des soins spéciaux pour une raison quelconque?

17. Les mères qui allaitent leur enfant reçoivent-elles de la documentation imprimée qui leur donne des indications et des informations?

Sortie

18. L'établissement a-t-il pour politique, si des "colis-cadeaux" contenant des produits destinés aux soins personnels de la mère et à ceux du nouveau-né sont remis aux mères lorsqu'elles sortent, de veiller à ce que ces colis ne contiennent rien qui risque de compromettre l'adoption et la poursuite de la pratique d'allaitement au sein, par exemple des biberons, des tétines, des sucettes ou des préparations pour nourrissons?

19. Les mères—ou d'autres membres de la famille le cas échéant—des enfants qui ne sont pas nourris au sein reçoivent-ils des indications adéquates conernant la préparation et l'administration correctes des substituts du lait maternel, et sont-ils mis en garde contre les risques pour la santé d'une mauvaise préparation?
    - L'établissement a-t-il pour politique de ne pas donner ces indications en présence de mères qui allaitent?

20. Toutes les mères reçoivent-elles un rendez-vous pour leur première visite de suivi en vue de bénéficier de soins postnatals et d'en faire donner à leur enfant?
    - Sont-elles informées de la façon de résoudre les problèmes que pourrait présenter entre temps l'allaitement au sein?

Studying the weaning process[a]

By "weaning process" is meant the *progressive* transfer of the infant from breast milk as the sole source of nourishment to the usual family diet. There are a number of reasons why it might be important to study weaning. For example, information may be needed to help plan a programme to improve children's nutritional status, and a first step would be to learn about how children are weaned. It can also be useful to know whether children's nutritional status can be improved by modifying weaning practices or to verify results when mothers adopt new practices. Knowledge about weaning can also be useful for evaluating the success of a given programme or activity in terms of its impact on nutritional status. It would be helpful to know, for example, whether weaning practices that were thought to be harmful to health and nutritional status have been changed, e.g., through a public information campaign, and whether this in fact has resulted in improved child well-being.

Defining study objectives

Whatever the purpose of the study, a first task is to define as clearly as possible the questions to be asked. They could include the following:

(1) *How do mothers in the community wean their children (e.g., age when weaning is started and ended, kinds of foods used, methods of preparation and feeding, amount of food given, and number of feeds per day)?* The focus will be on usual practices but will also explore seasonal variations and changes introduced when children are ill.

(2) *To what extent do different weaning practices affect the health and nutritional status of children?* Some practices facilitate the transition from breast milk to the usual family diet; others can increase the likelihood that children become ill and malnourished, e.g., delayed introduction of solid foods, too abrupt or early a shift from breast milk to other foods, and feeding contaminated foods. A general survey of community weaning practices may provide information suggesting associations between various practices and child health problems. Epidemiological techniques like case–control or cohort studies will be

particularly useful in studying these associations in an attempt to isolate genuine risk factors related to the weaning process.

(3) *What influences the way mothers wean their children?* It is important to know the range of practices that mothers adopt and to have an adequate amount of accurate background information about the conditions under which children are weaned in order to develop ideas about the influences that are likely to affect weaning.

(4) *If the influences that appear to determine weaning practices are changed, do the practices themselves also change?* For example, mothers who have little or no formal education may be more likely to give their children less nutritious foods than mothers who have attended school. Is this a result of differences in education or is it linked to the economic capacity of individual mothers to buy more nutritious foods?

(5) *If weaning practices are changed, does the health and nutritional status of children improve?* To answer this question an experimental study and a control group are required. Children weaned on the basis of new practices have to be compared with a control group whose weaning practices remain unchanged.

(6) *Has the programme, established with the objective of changing the way children are weaned, been effective?* If it is suspected that particular weaning practices are harmful to child health and nutritional status, a programme may be designed to change them. In due course both the investigator and the programme sponsor will want to know whether or not the programme is actually succeeding in changing practices and to what effect.

(7) *Has the programme also led to changes in the health and nutritional status of the community's children?* Assuming that mothers have altered the way they wean their children, it will be useful to determine whether the effort put into changing these practices has been worthwhile. Perhaps other factors, e.g., infectious disease, have a stronger influence on child health than do weaning practices. Alternatively, a change in practices may indirectly lead to a worsening of child health, e.g., an earlier introduction of semi-solid foods could increase the incidence of diarrhoeal diseases.

Undertaking a study as part of a field programme

Studies of child feeding practices are more usually undertaken by persons who are already involved in community health or nutrition programmes than as part of isolated research activities. There are many advantages to this arrangement since resident

[a] Adapted from: **Nabarro, D. et al.** *Finding out how children are weaned: guidelines prepared for staff of health, nutrition and development programmes who want to find out more about weaning practices and their possible consequences for children's well-being.* Unpublished document NUT/83.1 Geneva, World Health Organization, 1983.

programme staff are inclined to ensure that the questions examined are directly relevant to their everyday work. They are also more likely than outside researchers to be known and trusted by the local population and to know and understand community practices. Programme staff are also well placed to collect data over long periods, while they are also able to continually update information from households as an integral part of a programme's routine activities.

Doing research in the context of health or development programmes is not without its disadvantages, however. Staff might be tempted to discard information that is not favourable to them, and they may find it particularly difficult to study a random sample or to collect data from a control group. Households omitted from a sample may be upset at missing out, while those selected may wonder what is so interesting about them. A study that has no apparent benefit for staff or local populations may be resented, especially if it takes up a lot of people's time when data have to be collected from control groups not served by a programme. Programme staff are unlikely to let data collection take precedence over their ordinary work.

Obtaining needed information

Once it has been decided what questions to ask, the next step is to work out the kinds of information needed to answer them. A description of the weaning patterns adopted by mothers could include: the age at which weaning is begun and completed; types of food given; the number of times each day children are fed; quantity of food and nutrients consumed; cost of foods; methods of preparation; how children are fed; time used to prepare and feed children; extent of food contamination; and the quality of child supervision.

Information will come from a variety of sources although greatest emphasis will be placed on that which is known to be reliable. Staff from community-based programmes, who have been trained in data collection, are often found to be the most valuable providers of good quality information. They are asked to help interpret the raw data produced by large sample surveys, which may appear at first to be more "scientific" because of the volume of numbers they yield. At the same time, however, they can conceal a great deal of vital detail that can only be provided by people who know the situation. Programme staff working in the community, and indeed community members themselves, are thus extremely valuable informants.

Exploring the consequences of weaning practices

After learning how children are weaned, the next step will be to examine how particular practices affect their health and nutritional status. For example, do children who are breast-fed for more than six months gain more weight than children who are not? Does weight gain depend on the types of food supplements children receive or on how many times a day they are fed? Is there any difference in the incidence of illness among children who are or are not breast-fed? To answer these questions it is necessary to examine associations between weaning practices and child health and nutritional status, which requires a range of information including the rate of growth of individual children (defined as increases in weight or height over time); the number of times children are ill during a specified period and the duration of illness; and the numbers of children in the population who die or become disabled.

Examining influences on the way mothers wean their children

The weaning practices adopted by mothers are affected by a host of influences, and one way of analysing their effect would be to group them under headings which correspond to various study disciplines. For example, biological influences would include the health of the child and the mother and the birth of a new child. Cultural influences would include traditional values and rituals, education and advertising. Economic influences would include a family's ability to produce enough food, or to earn enough money to buy it, and the demands on a mother's time affecting her ability to prepare it for her family.

In reality, of course, influences on weaning practices operate together, and thus it might be preferable to group them in terms of the level at which they act. Five levels are identified for this purpose: the individual child, the individual mother, the mother–child unit, the household, and the community or nation.

At the level of the child, the influences are a direct result of bodily functions, including appetite, alterations in nutrient availability and illness. Other influences operate at the level of the child's mother and include her knowledge and beliefs about her child's nutritional needs, her experience and skills in feeding and caring for her child, and her own health and nutritional status. A third level considers the family as a whole, examining weaning practices in the context of available resources and the demands that all family members, including economically unproductive members, make on these resources and the impact of the views of important family members (authority figures). A fourth level is concerned with economic and political relationships in the community and understanding how they influence both the resources available to the household unit and the

Fig 1. A framework for examining the individual child, household and community influences on the way mothers wean their children.

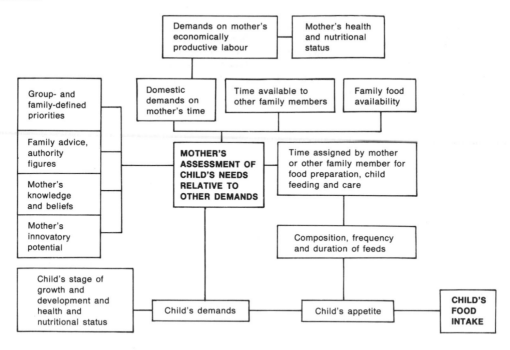

way these resources are used. A fifth and final level considers the nutritional problems of children from a national and international perspective, focusing on how relationships between countries influence infant- and child-feeding patterns. All but the last level of this framework for examining the influences on the way mothers wean their children are set out in Fig. 1.

Evaluating the effectiveness and impact of programmes

There will probably be a number of programmes operating in the community whose aim is to promote the general social and economic welfare or provide basic services for particular groups, for example health care for mothers and children. These programmes need to be systematically examined and their results assessed, and answers to the following questions may be useful for this purpose:

- What does the programme do and what is it trying to achieve?
- Who has access to the services provided and who actually uses them?
- How are the services used?
- Has the programme had a positive impact on the community's well-being?

Depending on the situation, it may be both unneces-

sary and a waste of resources to look for evidence of a programme's impact on the health and nutritional status of children. For example, if the level of services provided is low and coverage of the target population or use of services provided is minimal, it is unlikely that the programme will have widespread impact.

Many items of information have been identified for use in studying child weaning, although clearly not all are necessary at the same time. In planning a study, if the questions for which answers will be sought are clearly defined, it will be easier to list the information that will be required to answer them. As understanding of the weaning process increases, the list of required information will be updated, gradually leading to a reduction of the final number of items required.

Building a model

In order to make sense of the information to be collected about weaning, it will be necessary to develop a model of the weaning process. The model will be modified over time, sometimes radically, to accommodate new information. A decision has to be made about the model's overall structure. Thinking about the general questions that are to be asked (part 1) can be facilitated by making use of what is already known about the weaning process to prepare a series of possible answers to initial questions. Details can be filled in under each of the points, which describe the circumstances governing the adoption of various practices, and consideration given to whether particular practices have adverse effects on the health and nutritional status of weaning-age children. A simple diagram might help (see Fig. 1), showing some of the possible links between influencing factors, practices adopted, and health or nutritional consequences for the child.

In the beginning all of the information that is needed to answer questions will not be available; details can be added along the way. Work should continue on the model in an attempt to predict which factors have greatest influence on practices adopted and which practices are most likely to affect the health and nutritional status of the weaning-age child. It may then be useful to add to the model the different kinds of health, nutrition and development activities that are thought to influence either the weaning practices that families adopt or the health and nutritional status of their children.

In designing the study, it is suggested that time should be devoted to putting the model together on paper with the help of diagrams and drawings. A record, too, should be kept of how the model changes. The model will be used to help decide which information items are required and how they will facilitate concentration on those weaning practices that are of greatest interest. Studies will be set up to test these parts of the model to see if they represent what happens in reality. The model becomes increasingly more comprehensive as more and more of the already available information is collected. The model in turn helps in the decision about what extra information may be needed.

Sources of information

While deciding on the general questions to be studied and the information that is required to answer them, it is important to determine whether any of the information is already available. Information may be obtained from past surveys on nutritional status, patterns of illness, food intakes, and death rates. If a community has never before been studied, the results of studies undertaken in similar environments may be of help. Results from anthropological and economic surveys may serve to identify various social and economic groups. Records of rainfall, crop yields, market prices, sales of food and agricultural inputs, and food imports and exports can be valuable sources of information. Universities, research institutes and national, regional and international offices of multilateral and bilateral development agencies may also prove helpful.

It will be worthwhile to discuss questions with people who are knowledgeable about the community and the problems to be studied. This includes community leaders, government officers, and managers and staff of the research team. Health workers, teachers, and agricultural extension agents, whose day-to-day work brings them into close contact with the community, may also serve as useful sources. The poor and disadvantaged normally have limited opportunities to put their views across, yet their experiences can provide a wealth of important information. The success of the study may well depend on the active interest and cooperation of the people seen during the early stages of investigation. Similarly, even a short period of on-the-spot observation might prove to be more useful than lengthy library research.

The importance of a multidisciplinary approach cannot be overemphasized. The skills and knowledge of one discipline are bound to be insufficient to study all aspects of a household's life-style that affect infant and child feeding. For example, an anthropologist might try to understand the meaning of food taboos as an extension of the beliefs and values of the people practising them. An economist might be valuable in understanding the feeding choices open to households based on resource availability. A historian might explore what happened in the past as one way of gauging the likelihood of new ideas being accepted today. Ideally, persons from a variety of disciplines will work together. If this is not possible, every effort should be made to understand and apply at least the basic principles of the most relevant disciplines that relate to the forces that shape people's everyday lives.

Organizing and planning a study of weaning practices

Before starting a study, a plan of what is intended to be done and when will have to be drawn up. This plan will indicate what resources are needed including personnel, supplies and equipment and how much they are expected to cost. Once the study is under way the plan will serve as a reminder of what needs to be done and when. Compromise may be necessary to keep within the allotted budget, for example limits on the geographical area to be covered or on the number of households to be studied.

When planning a study it is important to consider all the different activities that are to be undertaken. Not only will a decision have to be made whether or not to collect all the data that are needed, but also whether it will be possible to convert these data into meaningful information and appropriate programme action. Merely collecting large amounts of data too easily leads to unexpected processing difficulties and a belated decision to analyse only a small portion. Results appearing after long delays are often out of date and are therefore of minimal value for re-programming purposes.

Even where resources are sufficient to prepare a large-scale study, it is strongly recommended that a small pilot study be undertaken first. However well prepared a study may be, there are bound to be some difficulties at each stage of its implementation. If a modest and manageable pilot study is first prepared to answer a number of basic questions, the chances of obtaining meaningful results later on will be enhanced. Some results can be obtained without major problems and the investigator and field workers will gain important experience. Many questions will remain unanswered but the pilot study will suggest other matters on which more information would be useful. A more detailed study can then be designed to include these as well.

After completing the pilot study, the next step will be to decide on the size and scope of the main study. Once again, available resources may prevent the undertaking of an "ideal" study and compromises will have to be made. For example, it may not be possible to undertake detailed analytical epidemiological surveys to explore relationships between individual influences and weaning practices, or between individual practices and health or nutritional consequences for the child. By using a case-study approach and carefully studying a small number of households, however, it should be possible to obtain a good idea of the conditions in which children are being weaned and the factors that combine to influence their health and nutritional status as a result.

Case studies can sometimes yield data that are difficult to process because of a failure to standardize them, while the number of cases is often small. Care has to be taken in applying the results of a case study to an entire population, especially if certain households have been deliberately chosen for study, because they may not be representative of the entire population group. On the other hand, despite the large amounts of data provided by sample surveys that can be readily processed into tables and graphs, in practice only limited conclusions can usually be drawn from them. It is impossible to collect and process data on every aspect of a household, although general statements may be made about influences on, or the possible consequences of, weaning practices in the population as a whole. At the same time, it is important to avoid oversimplifying the complexities of people's lives by trying to express everything in numbers.

Whether it is a question of incorporating data collection into the regular activities of a development programme or setting up a special study, a brief but comprehensive study plan should be prepared. The plan's *introduction* should include details about the purpose of the study and the specific questions it sets out to examine. The *methods* section should spell out the data that are to be collected, households or individuals from whom data are to be obtained, and the frequency of data collection activities. A section on *personnel* should list the staff required together with desirable qualifications, short job descriptions and training requirements. A part dealing with *administration* should include anticipated transportation, accommodation, meals, computing and other needs. The plan should include a *timetable* specifying the likely scheduling of the different phases of data collection, analysis and reporting.

The detailed design of data collection should not be undertaken without the help of the field workers who are responsible for collecting the data. These workers may know the study area and may even have done the same type of study before; if so, they will be invaluable sources of information and advice about questions to examine, information to obtain, and groups to study.

Field workers require special skills when case-study approaches are used. They will be expected not only to collect quantitative data, but also to obtain detailed information about attitudes and opinions underlying behaviour. Team leaders and supervisors capable of assuming responsibility for particular tasks will also be required. In a study carried out in the context of a health or development programme, data will often be collected by the programme staff, which may prove to be an advantage. There are other circumstances, however, where outsiders may be able to collect more, and more accurate, data than local staff, for example those associated with an unpopular institution.

The amount of time spent on training field workers will be determined largely by the scale of the study that is being undertaken, the size of the team, workers' previous experience, and the range of methods and data collection instruments to be used. Supervisors require personal experience with the data collection techniques that are to be used before they can instruct others in their application. Field workers need to be carefully trained in interview techniques so that they can produce data that are easily manipulated while causing little inconvenience to respondents, and to reduce errors to a minimum.

Five stages may be identified in a training programme for field workers. The *first* stage is an explanation of the purpose of the investigation. From the start, field workers should be invited to contribute their knowledge, ideas and experience and, in particular, to assist with the wording of the questions to be asked. During the *second* stage, trainees should begin to practise data collection on their own. Role-playing is an invaluable tool for providing participants an opportunity to interview and observe respondents with sensitivity and care, while they build up their confidence and skills in interviewing techniques. The *third* stage of training is the supervised interview under the unobtrusive eye of the trainer, who monitors the interaction between worker and respondent and checks the quality of the data obtained. The *fourth* stage consists of practice interviews conducted in a number of test households, which can be made even more valuable if recorded by voice or, better still, video tape. The *fifth*, and most important, stage of training has new field workers teaming up with others more experienced in such surveys in order to continue their apprenticeship and gain the necessary confidence that only practice can bring.

Whether for a large-scale field survey or for a small-scale case study, proper management is required to ensure that data are collected, the work is completed within the budgetary and time limits, and the study causes no disturbance in the community. Survey managers responsible for data collection will need to manage the flow of data as well as resources allotted for their collection. Field workers' data collection tasks should be clearly set out and accomplished on schedule. Data will have to be checked on arrival for any errors and bias, and particular attention will have to be paid to correcting the source of any problems in cooperation with field workers. Communication between all members of the survey team has to be maintained, including rapid feedback on any problems that may have occurred and the provisional results of the survey.

Accounting systems will have to be set up to handle cash flow. Project backers will wish to have an accurate accounting of how their money was spent. It will also be necessary to review whether time, staff and materials are being used to maximum efficiency. Studies of weaning practices require close contact between field workers and households in the population under study. A vital requirement, in order to avoid misunderstandings, is an efficient system for communicating plans, ideas and needs between the survey team, community members, project backers and the study manager.

It is also necessary to establish and maintain rapport with people in the community who are not participating in the survey, and who may be concerned about what is happening or how the survey results will be used. Influential persons should be consulted and the study's purpose and results explained to them. However, an effort should be made to communicate with all sections of the community and not just those persons in positions of authority.

The quality of the survey also depends on the morale and motivation of field workers. Re-training sessions at regular intervals during the study may help to provide both motivation and encouragement.

Résumé
Comment étudier le processus de sevrage

Par sevrage il faut entendre le passage progressif pour un nourrisson du lait maternel comme aliment unique au régime alimentaire familial habituel. L'étude du sevrage est importante à plus d'un titre, notamment dans la planification et l'évaluation de programmes destinés à améliorer l'état nutritionnel des enfants.

Définition des objectifs de l'étude

Dans une première étape les questions à poser pourraient être les suivantes:

1. Comment dans une communauté les mères sèvrent-elles leurs enfants?
2. Dans quelle mesure les pratiques de sevrage peuvent-elles affecter l'état de santé et l'état nutritionnel des enfants?
3. Quels sont les éléments qui influencent la manière dont les mères sèvrent leurs enfants?
4. Si ces influences changent, est-ce que les pratiques changent aussi?
5. Si les pratiques de sevrage changent, est-ce que l'état sanitaire et nutritionnel des enfants s'améliore?
6. Un programme a été établi avec pour objectif de modifier la manière dont les enfants sont sevrés. A-t-il été efficace?
7. Est-ce que ce programme a amené des modifications dans l'état nutritionnel et de santé des enfants de la communauté?

Mise en œuvre de l'enquête dans le cadre d'un programme de terrain

Il y a beaucoup d'avantages à utiliser les personnels de terrain pour conduire des recherches, aussi bien du point de vue de la pertinence que de celui de l'acceptabilité locale. Les désavantages résident dans le fait que certaines informations jugées défavorables peuvent ne pas être transmises. Le bénéfice de la recherche peut ne pas être apparent et surtout le travail quotidien peut ne laisser que peu de place aux enquêtes.

Cadre conceptuel pour analyser les influences qu'exercent l'enfant, le foyer et la communauté sur la façon dont les mères sèvrent leurs nourrissons.

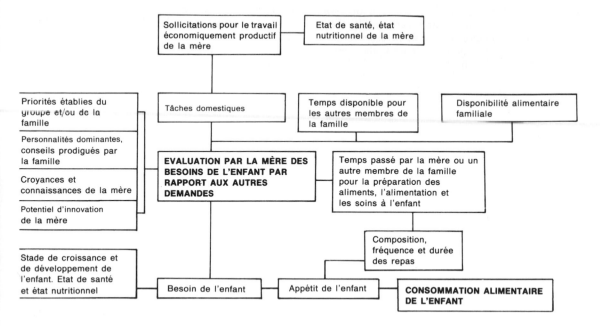

Recueillir l'information nécessaire

L'étape suivante consiste à recueillir certains types d'informations à des sources nombreuses et diverses:

— âge auquel le sevrage débute et celui auquel il est achevé;
— types d'aliments offerts et nombre de repas par jour;
— quantité d'aliments ingérés, coût et méthodes de préparation;
— manière dont les enfants sont alimentés, temps passé à les préparer et à les nourrir;
— importance de la contamination des aliments;
— qualité de la surveillance de l'enfant.

Examen des conséquences des pratiques de sevrage

Au cours de l'étape suivante on examinera comment certaines pratiques affectent l'état de santé et l'état nutritionnel des enfants. Par exemple: après 6 mois comment évolue le poids des enfants qui sont toujours au sein par rapport à ceux qui ne le sont pas? Quelle est l'importance de la morbidité et de la mortalité dans la population infantile objet de l'étude?

Examen des facteurs qui déterminent la manière dont les mères sèvrent leurs enfants

Les influences qui interviennent sont nombreuses et il vaudrait mieux les regrouper sous des rubriques différentes: biologiques, culturelles, économiques. Dans la réalité les interactions sont multiples, il est préférable de les étudier selon des niveaux différents: l'enfant, la mère, le couple mère-enfant, le foyer, la communauté ou la nation. Tous ces niveaux, à part le dernier, sont analysés dans leur inter-relations dans le cadre développé ci-dessus (voir figure).

Dans ce cadre de recherche sur le sevrage sont aussi considérés les points suivants:

— l'évaluation de l'efficacité et de l'impact des programmes;
— l'élaboration d'un modèle;
— les sources d'information;
— l'organisation et la planification d'une étude du processus de sevrage.

ANNEX 3

Suggested further reading

Selected WHO publications (prices in US$)

Aldrin and dieldrin. Environmental Health Criteria, No. 91. 1989 (335 pages), ISBN 92 4 154291 8, $30.60.

Contemporary patterns of breast-feeding. Report on the WHO Collaborative Study on Breast-feeding. 1981 (211 pages), ISBN 92 4 156067 3, $21.60.

Jelliffe, D.B. & Jelliffe, E.F.P. *Dietary management of young children with diarrhoea. A practical manual for district programme managers.* 1989 (28 pages), ISBN 92 4 154246 2, $7.20. Revised edition in preparation.

DDT and its derivatives. Environmental Health Criteria, No. 9. 1979 (194 pages), ISBN 92 4 154069 9, $14.40.

Energy and protein requirements. Report of a Joint FAO/WHO/UNU Expert Consultation. WHO Technical Report Series, No. 724. 1985 (206 pages), ISBN 92 4 120724 8, $15.30.

The growth chart. A tool for use in infant and child health care. 1986 (33 pages), ISBN 92 4 154208 X, $10.80.

Beghin, I., Cap, M. & Dujardin, B. *A guide to nutritional assessment.* 1988 (80 pages), ISBN 92 4 154221 7, $12.60.

Guidelines for training community health workers in nutrition. Second edition 1986 (121 pages), ISBN 92 4 154210 1, $14.40.

Having a baby in Europe. Report on a study. Public Health in Europe, No. 26. 1985 (157 pages), ISBN 92 890 1162 9, $11.70.

James, W.P.T. et al. *Healthy nutrition. Preventing nutrition-related diseases in Europe.* 1988 (150 pages), ISBN 92 890 1115 7, $18.00.

Iodine-deficiency disorders in South-East Asia. SEARO Regional Health Papers, No. 10. 1985 (96 pages), ISBN 92 9022 179 8, $6.30.

The management of diarrhoea and use of oral rehydration therapy. A Joint WHO/UNICEF Statement. Second edition. 1985 (25 pages), ISBN 92 4 156086 X, $2.70.

Maternal care for the reduction of perinatal and neonatal mortality. A Joint WHO/UNICEF Statement. 1986 (22 pages), ISBN 92 4 156099 1, $2.70.

Measuring change in nutritional status. Guidelines for assessing the nutritional impact of supplementary feeding programmes for vulnerable groups. 1983 (101 pages), 92 4 154166 0, $12.60.

Minor and trace elements in breast milk. Report of a Joint WHO/IAEA Collaborative Study. 1989 (171 pages), ISBN 92 4 156121 1, $27.00.

Nutrition learning packages. Joint WHO/UNICEF Nutrition Support Programme. 1989 (170 pages), ISBN 92 4 154 251 9, $27.00.

Gopalan, C. *Nutrition—problems and programmes in South-East Asia.* SEARO Regional Health Papers, No. 15. 1987 (174 pages), ISBN 92 9022 184 4, $15.30.

Mason, J.B. et al. *Nutritional surveillance.* 1984 (194 pages), ISBN 92 4 156078 9, $20.70.

Prenatal and perinatal infections. EURO Reports and Studies, No. 93. 1985 (147 pages), ISBN 92 890 1259 5, $10.80.

DeMaeyer, E. et al. *Preventing and controlling iron deficiency anaemia through primary health care. A guide for health administrators and programme managers.* 1989 (58 pages), ISBN 92 4 154249 7, $9.90

Prevention in childhood and youth of adult cardiovascular diseases. Time for action. Report of a WHO Expert Committee. WHO Technical Report Series No. 792, 1990 (105 pages), ISBN 92 4 120792 2, $10.80.

Protecting, promoting and supporting breast-feeding. The special role of maternity services. A Joint WHO/UNICEF Statement. 1989 (32 pages), ISBN 92 4 156130 0, $5.40.

The quantity and quality of breast milk. Report on the WHO Collaborative Study on Breast-feeding. 1985 (148 pages), ISBN 92 4 154201 2, $15.30.

Selenium. Environmental Health Criteria, No. 58. 1987 (306 pages), ISBN 92 4 154258 6, $21.60.

Treatment and prevention of acute diarrhoea. Practical guidelines. Second edition. 1989 (54 pages), ISBN 92 4 154243 8, $9.90.

Vitamin A supplements. A guide to their use in the treatment and prevention of vitamin A deficiency and xerophthalmia. 1988 (24 pages), ISBN 92 4 154236 5, $7.20.

Weaning—from breast milk to family food. A guide for health and community workers. 1988 (36 pages), ISBN 92 4 154237 3, $8.10.

Further information on these and other WHO publications can be obtained from Distribution and Sales, World Health Organization, 1211 Geneva 27, Switzerland.

Other publications

Lawrence, R.A. *Breast-feeding: A guide for the medical profession.* Saint Louis: C.V. Mosby Co. 1989.

Renfrew, M.J., Fisher, C. & Arms, S. *Bestfeeding: getting breastfeeding right for you.* Berkeley, California: Celestial Arts, 1990.

Minchin, M.K. *Breastfeeding matters: what we need to know about infant feeding.* Melbourne: Alma Publications, 1989.

Chalmers, I., Enkin, M.W., Kierse, M.J.N.C. (ed.). *Effective care in pregnancy and childbirth.* Chapters 21, 80, 81 & 89. Oxford: Oxford University Press, 1989.

Francis, D.E.M. *Diets for sick children.* Oxford: Blackwell Scientific Publications, 1987.

Bennett P.N. & the WHO Working Group. *Drugs and human lactation.* Amsterdam: Elsevier, 1988.

Jensen, R.G. & Neville, M.C. *Human lactation: milk components and methodologies.* New York: Plenum Press, 1985.

Hamosh, M. & Goldman, A. (ed.) *Human lactation 2: maternal and environmental factors.* New York: Plenum Press, 1986.

Goldman, A.S., Atkinson, S.A. & Hanson, L.A. (ed.). *Human lactation 3: effects on the recipient infant.* New York: Plenum Press, 1987.

Howell, R.R., Morriss, F.H. & Pickering, L.K. *Human milk in infant nutrition and health.* Springfield: C.C. Thomas, 1986.

Jelliffe, D.B. & Jelliffe, E.F.P. *Human milk in the modern world.* Oxford: Oxford University Press, 1978 (revised edition in preparation).

Williams, A.F. & Baum, J.D. *Human milk banking.* New York: Raven Press, 1984.

Hanson L. *The immunology of the neonate.* Berlin: Springer Verlag, 1988.

Tsang, R.C. & Nichols, B.L. *Nutrition during infancy.* Saint Louis: C.V. Mosby Co., 1988.

Jelliffe, D.B. & Jelliffe, E.F.P. *Programmes to promote breast-feeding.* Oxford: Oxford University Press, 1988.

Chandra, R.K. (ed.). *Trace elements in the nutrition of children.* New York: Raven Press, 1985.

Information and resources materials

American Public Health Association, 1015 Fifteenth Street, N.W., Washington, DC 20005, USA.

Appropriate Health Resources and Technology Action Group (AHRTAG), 1 London Bridge Street, London SE1 9SG, England.

Center for Breast-feeding Information, La Leche League International, 9616 Minneapolis Avenue, Franklin Park, Illinois 60131, USA.

Lactation Resource Centre, Nursing Mothers Association of Australia, P.O. Box 231, Nunawading 3131, Victoria, Australia.

Midwives Information and Resource Service, Institute of Child Health, Royal Hospital for Sick Children, Saint Michael's Hill, Bristol BS2 8BJ, England.

Oxford Database of Perinatal Trials, National Perinatal Epidemiology Unit, Radcliffe Infirmary, Oxford, England.

TALC (Teaching Aids at Low Cost), P.O. Box 49, Saint Albans, Herts. AL1 4AX, England.

PROTECTING, PROMOTING AND SUPPORTING
BREAST-FEEDING

The special role of maternity services

A Joint WHO/UNICEF Statement

■ Breast-feeding is an unequalled way of providing ideal food for the healthy growth and development of infants and has a unique biological and emotional influence on the health of both mother and child.

■ In extreme cases, whole generations of young mothers have never seen a woman breast-feed and know nothing about a practice that they consider old-fashioned and no longer necessary.

■ Often, procedures and routines are introduced for seemingly valid scientific and organzational reasons, or for the convenience of the health care staff in providing what are perceived as efficient and effective services. Rarely is thought given to the implications of these procedures and routines for breast-feeding practice.

■ The fact that so many infants currently leave hospitals and clinics already bottle-fed is contributing considerably to the decline in the prevalence of breast-feeding. Only small quantities of breast-milk substitutes are ordinarily required in health care facilities for the few infants who cannot be breast-fed.

■ While discoveries are still being made about the many benefits of breast milk and breast-feeding, few today would openly contest the maxim "breast is best". Yet slogans, however accurate, are no substitute for action.

■ WHO and UNICEF believe that health care practices, particularly those related to the care of mothers and newborn infants, stand out as one of the most promising means of increasing the prevalence and duration of breast-feeding.

Protecting, Promoting and Supporting Breast-feeding: The Special Role of Maternity Services 1989, iv + 32 pages, ISBN 92 4 156130 0 (Available in Arabic, English, French and Spanish; *see Annex 1 for list of other languages in preparation*) Sw.fr, 6,–/US $5 40

- -

DSA.MCH.90.A

Order form

☐ Please send me ____ copy/ies of **Protecting, Promoting and Supporting Breast-feeding** at Sw.fr. 6.–/US $5.40 per copy (1150326)

☐ Payment enclosed

☐ Please charge to my credit card

   ☐ Visa   ☐ American Express
   ☐ Eurocard/Mastercard/Access

Card number

Expiry date   Date of order

Signature

Name

Address

Return to WHO at the address listed below. Special rates for bulk purchase are available on request.

WHO • Distribution and Sales • 1211 Geneva 27 • Switzerland

PROTECTION, ENCOURAGEMENT ET SOUTIEN DE L'ALLAITEMENT MATERNEL

Le rôle spécial des services liés à la maternité

Déclaration conjointe de l'OMS et de l'UNICEF

■ L'allaitement au sein constitue un moyen sans égal de nourrir l'enfant de la façon qui convient le mieux pour sa croissance et son bon développement et il exerce en outre une influence biologique et affective sans pareille sur l'état de santé de la mère et de l'enfant.

■ Dans les cas extrêmes, des générations entières de jeunes mères n'ont jamais vu une femme allaiter son enfant et ne savent rien d'une pratique qu'elles considèrent comme démodée et dépourvue désormais de toute nécessité.

■ Il arrive souvent que ces services adoptent telles ou telles procédures et pratiques pour des raisons scientifiques ou organisationnelles apparemment valables, ou bien pour permettre à leurs personnels d'assurer commodément ce qu'ils considèrent comme des prestations à la fois productives et efficaces. Il est rare que l'on pense aux conséquences que ces procédures et pratiques peuvent avoir sur le plan de l'allaitement maternel.

■ La diminution de la prévalence de l'allaitement maternel tient pour beaucoup au fait que beaucoup de nourrissons quittent actuellement l'hôpital ou la clinique déjà nourris au biberon. Les établissements de soins n'ont en général besoin que de faibles quantités de substituts du lait maternel pour les quelques nouveau-nés que l'on ne peut nourrir au sein.

■ Si l'on découvre toujours de nouveaux avantages venant s'ajouter à ceux, déjà nombreux, du lait maternel et de l'allaitement au sein, rares sont ceux qui aujourd'hui pourraient contester ouvertement le slogan "le sein, c'est plus sain". Pourtant, les slogans, même s'ils correspondent étroitement à la réalité, ne sauraient se substituer à l'action.

■ L'OMS et l'UNICEF estiment que, les prestations sanitaires, et notamment celles dispensées aux mères et aux nouveau-nés, constituent l'un des moyens les plus prometteurs d'accroître la prévalence et la durée de cette pratique.

Protection, encouragement et soutien de l'allaitement maternel. Le rôle spécial des services liés à la maternité
1989, iv + 32 pages, ISBN 92 4 256130 4
(Disponible en arabe, anglais, français et espagnol; voir l'annexe 1 pour les autres langues en préparation)
Fr.s. 6.–/US $5.40

Bulletin de commande

DSA.MCH.90.1.F

☐ Veuillez m'envoyer ——— exemplaire(s) de **Protection, encouragement et soutien de l'allaitement maternel** au prix de Fr.s. 6.—/ US $5.40 l'exemplaire (2150326)

☐ Paiement joint

☐ Veuillez débiter ma carte de crédit

   ☐ Visa   ☐ American Express
   ☐ Eurocard/Mastercard/Access

N° de carte _____

Date d'expiration _____ Date de commande _____

Signature _____

Nom _____

Adresse _____
_____
_____
_____

Renvoyer à l'adresse ci-dessous. Demander nos tarifs spéciaux pour les commandes en quantité.

OMS · Distribution et Ventes · 1211 Genève 27 · Suisse

VIENT DE PARAITRE

Alimentation infantile
Bases physiologiques

La présente publication établit les bases scientifiques qui permettent d'aborder les nombreuses questions relatives à l'alimentation appropriée de l'enfant durant la première année de sa vie. Notant qu'un régime adéquat est plus décisif au cours des premières années qu'à un autre moment de la vie, l'étude considère que les connaissances acquises en matière de physiologie du nourrisson peuvent contribuer à mieux comprendre les besoins nutritionnels. On trouvera ci-joint plus de 500 références à cette littérature. Outre qu'elles confirment les avantages uniques du lait maternel, qui reste la seule vraie source universelle de nutrition du nourrisson, les données examinées remettent en cause certaines hypothèses couramment émises, comme les circonstances où s'imposent les préparations pour nourrissons disponibles dans le commerce, le meilleur moment pour introduire l'alimentation de complément et le régime alimentaire le mieux adapté aux nourrissons de petits poids de naissance.

L'ouvrage est divisé en six chapitres principaux. Le premier, consacré aux périodes prénatale et du postpartum, examine les mécanismes physiologiques qui entrent en jeu pendant la grossesse, déterminent les besoins énergétiques de la mère, affectent la croissance foetale et régissent les besoins nutritionnels du nourrisson. De plus, il fait le résumé des récentes preuves scientifiques qui militent en faveur de l'importance du contact mère-enfant immédiatement après la naissance. Le deuxième chapitre traite de la physiologie de la lactation et donne un compte rendu fascinant des mécanismes complexes qui préparent le sein à la lactation, gouvernent la lactogenèse et le maintien de la lactation, préparent le nourrisson à l'allaitement au sein, protègent le sein et contribuent à la santé maternelle. Par ailleurs, ce chapitre examine les mécanismes grâce auxquels le lait maternel apporte une protection contre l'infec-tion et les allergies et explique pourquoi les concentrations du lait maternel en protéines, matières grasses, lactose, vitamines, minéraux et oligo-éléments sont très précisément les seules qui soient indiquées pour satisfaire les besoins de la croissance du nourrisson et augmenter sa capacité métabolique.

Les facteurs pouvant interférer avec l'allaitement au sein sont examinés au troisième chapitre, qui traite des cas de nourrissons présentant des troubles congénitaux ou héréditaires du métabolisme, bec de lièvre ou fentes palatines, ainsi que différentes maladies de la mère, y compris l'infection au VIH. Dans ce chapitre, il est expliqué pourquoi le lait maternel reste la source de nutrition la plus appropriée dans presque tous les cas où l'enfant ou la mère sont en mauvaise santé. Le quatrième chapitre examine la question cruciale de l'alimentation de complément. Il y est dit en conclusion que le lait maternel satisfait à lui seul les besoins énergétiques d'un nourrisson normal au cours des six premiers mois de la vie et qu'une alimentation de complément précoce peut entraîner un certain nombre de risques à court et à long termes. Les autres chapitres examinent les besoins spécifiques de deux groupes particulièrement vulnérables : les nourrissons de petits poids de naissance et les nourrissons et jeunes enfants atteints de maladies infectieuses.

Alimentation infantile
Bases physiologiques
Publié sous la direction de *J. Akré*
Organisation mondiale de la Santé, 1992
environ 100 pages (anglais, français, espagnol)
ISBN 92 4 068671 1
Francs suisses : 20.-- (N° de commande 2036701)
Prix dans les pays en développement : Fr.s. 14.--

Organisation mondiale de la Santé · Distribution et Vente · 1211 Genève 27 · Suisse

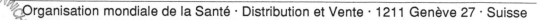